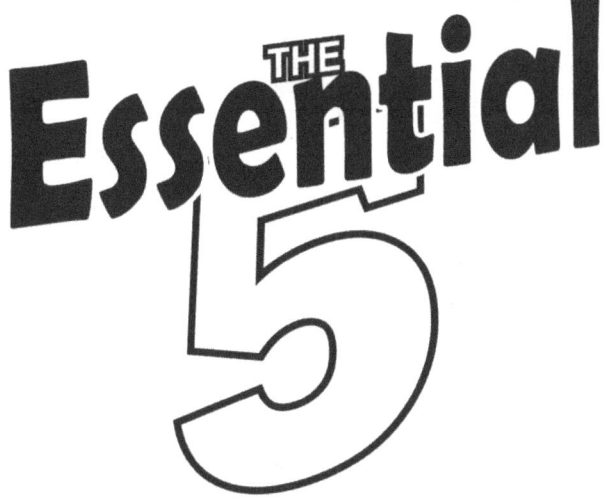

Make Your OWN Natural Products using only FIVE Essential Oils or Less

Over 200 Easy and Effective Recipes

Tina Fletcher

The Essential 5:
How to Make Natural Products Using 5 Essential Oils or Less

Author: Tina Fletcher

PO Box 478
AYR Queensland 4807
Australia

A.B.N. 14 025 759 182

www.TheEssential5.com
Email: tina@tinafletcher.com

Copyright © Tina Fletcher

First Published by Tina Fletcher Designs in January 2010

Tina Fletcher asserts the moral right to be identified as the author of this work.

All rights reserved. No part of the publication may be reproduced, in whole or in part, stored in a retrieval system, posted on the internet or transmitted, in any form or by any means, electronic, mechanical, photocopying, recording or otherwise, without prior permission of the publishers or the author of the book.

IMPORTANT NOTICE
This book contains information on Essential Oils and Base Oils. It is intended as an information guide for your use, not as a medical reference book. Consult your doctor before replacing any existing medication with an aromatherapy treatment. The reader is advised not to self-treat for serious or long term problems without consulting with a qualified health practitioner. The material in this book is not meant to take the place of diagnosis and treatment. All recommendations herein contained are believed to be effective, but since the use of Essentials Oils is beyond the author's control, no expressed or implied guarantee is given as to the effect of their use. No liability is taken and the use of any Essential Oil is entirely at the reader's own risk.

ISBN 0980 785 901

*This book is dedicated to
My wonderful children,
Cassie, Jade, Lachlan, Gabrielle and Thomas
who daily allow me to appreciate
the true meaning of success.*

Contents

Acknowledgement 8
Preface 9

Introduction 11
    Terms to Remember 13

SECTION 1
The Essential 5 15
    Why Five Essential Oils 16
    Additional Essential Oils Needed for Perfume 19
    Why have Starter Kits 20
    The Cost Benefits of using Essential Oils 21

SECTION 2
The Wonders of Essential Oils 23
    Enjoying the benefits of Essentials Oils 24
    Buying Essential Oils 26
    Looking after Your Oils 28
    The Top, the Middle and the Base of Essential Oil Notes 29
    Why Different Oils Have Different Prices 31
    Cautions Using Essential Oils 32

SECTION 3
Bases - Bringing It All Together 33
    Understanding the Need for Base Oils and Base Products 34
    Commonly use Base Oils and Their Properties 35
    How to Mix and Use Essential Oils with Bases 42

SECTION 4
Making Your Own 43
    So You Want To Make Your Own Products 44
    Effective Applications —Using your products 45
    Bottles and Jars: What's Best 48
    Creating Labels: Without Them, You Would Be Lost 49

SECTION 5
House Cleaning Naturally 51
How to Benefit at Home 53
The Cost Comparison of Your Household Cleaning Starter Kit 54
RECIPES: Household Cleaning Starter Kit 56
RECIPES: A-Z of Household Cleaning Product 67

SECTION 6
First Aid and Common Ailments Solutions 97
The Benefits of Natural First Aid Products 98
The Cost Comparison of Your First Aid Starter Kit 99
RECIPES: First Aid and Common Ailment starter Kit 100
Using Other Essential Oils 123
RECIPES: A-Z Common Ailments Products   Using Other Essential Oils 124

SECTION 7
Relaxation and Stress Relief Remedies 137
The Benefit of Relaxation and Stress Relief 141
The Cost Comparison of Your Relaxation and Stress Relief Kit 142
Relaxation and Stress Relief Essential 4 Blends 144
Effective Applications for You 145
Recipes: 5 Product Relaxation and Stress Relief Starter Kit 152
RECIPES: A-Z of Relaxation and Stress Relief 157

SECTION 8 163
Skin Care Sensations 163
The Benefits of Chemical-Free Skincare 164
The Cost Comparison of Your Skin Care Starter Kit 167
RECIPES: Skin Care Starter Kit 168
RECIPES: A-Z of Skincare 173

SECTION 9
Hair Care Help 181
The Benefits of looking after Your Crowning Glory naturally 183
The Cost Comparison of Your Hair Care Starter Kit 186
RECIPES: 5-Product Hair Care Starter Kit 187
RECIPES: A- Z of Hair Care 192

SECTION 10
Perfume Pampering 207
The Benefits of Your Own Perfume Blends 210
Perfumery's Essential 4 211
perfume and their aromatic notes 212
The Cost Comparison of your Perfume Starter Kit 213
Perfumery Layering System 214
Perfume Blend Using Essential 4 oils 215
Using Other Essential Oils to Create More Perfume Ranges 216
RECIPES: Perfume Starter Kit 217
RECIPES: A-Z of Perfumery Products 223

SECTION 11
Gorgeous Gift Ideas 231
Love Giving Gifts That Delight 232
A-Z of Gift Ideas 233

SECTION 12
Aromatherapy 243
What Is Aromatherapy 244
Aromatherapy History 246
How Essential Oils Are Made 248
Essential Oil Properties 249
A-Z Essential Oils 250

Conclusion 287
Conclusion 288
Biography 289
Index 291

ACKNOWLEDGEMENT

Thank you to all my wonderful friends, family and clients who have used these recipes and helped me fine tune them. Without their feedback and comments, this book would not be filled with so many great recipes and hints.

In the course of my aromatherapy studies, I have time and time again referred to several books and would like to acknowledge them here. Without their invaluable information, I would have taken longer to learn and discover the wonderful joy of using aromatherapy every day.

Valerie Ann Worwood, *The Fragrant Pharmacy*, published 1990

Nerys Purchon, *Handbook of Aromatherapy*, published 1999

Health and Harmony College, course notes for Advance Diploma in Aromatherapy and Diploma in Natural Beauty Therapy.

PREFACE

I wanted chemical-free, natural products made with simple step-by-step recipes. I wanted my own products that would benefit me, my family, and my friends. I have been using Essential Oils for years and I knew I could make effective products.

So, I started putting together all my recipes, I worked out the cost to make them and compare it to buying the equivalent products. I was right not only did I save money; I created products that work efficiently and smelled divine.

Lots of my friends and clients started using these recipes and Essential Oils for themselves and loved them. They found making their own wasn't hard and enjoyed the benefits of saving money while making natural products that were chemical free and smelled wonderful. I was asked time and time again for more products that they could make.

Creating a book on how to make natural products seemed inevitable.

We all agreed using Essential Oils and aromatherapy recipes was wonderful but sometimes found we had to buy lots of different oils to create a single product and sometime we never used up all of the Essential Oils we bought (this made it expensive). What if we could create them with fewer Essential Oils?

So one day after a few drinks and snacks, the idea was created—not only to write the book but to create recipes that used the same oils in different quantities and different ratios to make as many products as I could.

Could it be done?

Yes, it could. *The Essential 5* was created.

INTRODUCTION

We want you to enjoy using Essential Oils and make your own products from recipes that are quick and simple.

By using only 5 Essential Oils, you keep the cost down but you don't make inferior products. I would never compromise the effectiveness of these recipes if they wouldn't work with the five Essential Oils.

Cost You Less. By reducing the number of Essential Oils and combining them with common household ingredients, you spend less, waste less, and are able to make more as you want it.

Starter Kits. Each section gives you with the most commonly used products along with a check list of ingredients, bottles, and all equipment needed to make the Starter Kit.

Cost Comparison. Each section compares the cost to buy the item at the store (cheapest generic) to the cost of making products with Essential Oils and household ingredients.

Simple Recipes. By keeping the recipes simple to prepare and easy to follow, you can save yourself time along with money using *The Essential 5* recipes.

It is amazing how simple but still effective these products are. They are easy to make, to store, and to make up quickly as you need them. *The Essential 5* has over 200 quick and easy recipes. The products are great for you, for your family, and for inexpensive gifts that look (and smell) a million dollars.

If you love natural, chemical-free products, then this book is for you. If you also love to save money, then this book is definitely for you.

– The Essential 5 –

If you love making your own products, you will love the simple step-by-step recipes.

Even if you have never blended a product before this book is design to give you the easy instruction and all the information you need to make you own products.

The Essential 5 contains great recipes for

- ✓ Household Cleaning
- ✓ First Cid and Common Ailments
- ✓ Relaxation and Stress Relief
- ✓ Skin Care
- ✓ Hair Care
- ✓ Perfumery
- ✓ Gift Ideas

You can read this book cover to cover, or you can simply go to the chapter you're interested in and begin creating your own all-natural products.

TERMS TO REMEMBER

Here are a couple of terms we will use throughout this book when talking about Essential Oils and aromatherapy.

- ✓ **Properties.** The attributes or characteristics of an ingredient (an Essential Oil, Base Oil, or household ingredient)

- ✓ **Notes.** The strength of the aroma or scent (how long it lasts in the air or on your skin)

- ✓ **Blend.** The mixing of a product (same as a recipe)

- ✓ **Recipe.** The mixing of ingredients to make a product

SECTION 1

The Essential 5

WHY FIVE ESSENTIAL OILS

When we first decided to create recipes with a smaller number of oils, we tested three, four, and five Essential Oil blends and found that five oils gave us the most versatility and best value for money.

When selecting our Essential Oils we tested and tested them until we found the best.

- **Value.** Why use expensive oil if a less expensive one will work just as well?
- **Versatility.** What oils have many benefits and uses?
- **Properties.** What oils have a larger range or properties and work the best with our bodies and environment?
- **Simplicity.** What are the more commonly known oils?
- **Practicality.** What oils are easy to find?

Did you know?

Synergy is the working together of two things to produce an effect greater than the sum of their individual effects

wordnetweb.princeton.edu/perl/webwn .

*In Aromatherapy, if you blend three or more Essential Oils, you get better than three times the benefits.
Great extra benefit with no extra work!*

– The Essential 5 –

Here is a quick summary of the 5 Essential Oils used from the most common used to less common used (For more information, refer to "A-Z Essential Oils").

1. Lavender Essential Oil
2. Geranium Essential Oil
3. Lemon Essential Oil
4. Chamomile Essential Oil
5. Tea Tree Essential Oil

Lavender Essential Oil

The most popular Essential Oil is Lavender. If you were going to buy one Essential Oil, then Lavender would be the one. It is used in all sections of *The Essential 5*. This amazing oil is one of the most useful of all essential oils. Lavender's properties include being an antiseptic, a relaxant, an antitoxin, useful for burns, a sedative, a tonic, and a deodorant to name a few. It blends well with most other oils. It is bridging oil for perfumes and has a very common aroma.

Geranium Essential Oil

Geranium Essential Oil has a strong herbaceous aroma with similar notes to the rose. This great all-around Essential Oil has therapeutic properties as an astringent, antiseptic, anti-depressant, tonic, antibiotic, and as an anti-infectious agent. It aids against travel sickness and assists with irritations associated with dermatitis, eczema, and psoriasis.

Lemon Essential Oil

Well-known for its clean refreshing aroma, Lemon Essential Oil has high anti-bacterial properties. On skin and hair it can be used for its cleansing effect as well as for its antiseptic properties because it is refreshing and cooling. Lemon may assist the ability to concentrate. The tart smell is commonly associated with cleanliness.

Chamomile Essential Oil

Chamomile Essential Oil is useful to treat aches and pains in muscles and joints. Treatment of symptoms of PMS with Chamomile is also beneficial especially when the symptoms are related to stress. It has a long tradition in herbal medicine; the flowers were used in many cures, including an herbal tea, during World War II. The strong aroma of chamomile is fruity and herbaceous and ideal for children and those with sensitive skins.

Tea Tree Essential Oil

Most of us have used or own Tea Tree Essential Oil. It is used in two sections and is best known as a very powerful immune stimulant. It can help to fight off infectious. Used as part of an inhalation, it can help with colds, measles, and sinusitis and viral infections. For skin and hair, Tea Tree has been used to combat acne, oily skin, head lice, and dandruff.

ADDITIONAL ESSENTIAL OILS NEEDED FOR PERFUME

Ylang Ylang Essential Oil

Used extensively in perfumes and cosmetics because of its intensely heady floral aroma, Ylang Ylang Essential Oil has a very sweet exotic scent. It is reputed to be an aphrodisiac and a powerful stimulant with euphoric properties. Use in two sections, it can be used as a sedative and has a regulating effect on the nervous system; it may be used as general cleaner for skin and hair.

Jasmine Essential Oil

When you think of exotic oils, you think of Jasmine Essential Oil. Its highly fragrant aroma is known for its aphrodisiac qualities and it can work as a sedative to assist in calming and reduction of stress. It is one of the most expensive Essential Oils, and many synthetic copies are used in perfumes. Because of the high price of Jasmine, alternative and less expensive oils may be used. For example, it can be found at 3 percent in jojoba oil with the same benefits and aroma (ideal for perfumery).

You can find more information about these oils and many more at the back of the book in "A-Z Essential Oils".

As you can see, these Essential Oils are very versatile and beneficial. They are a great start for your journey to having fun and benefiting from the use of Essential Oils and aromatherapy.

WHY HAVE STARTER KITS

We have made Starter Kits for all sections. These will identify the most common products used and give you a place to start if you have never made your own products. You can also compare costs.

Each Starter Kit has been created by asking friends, clients and others about the products they would use the most and would like to have made up for daily or common use. We used questionnaires to survey online, at markets and in mail outs to gather responses.

We assessed this information and collated the Top 10 or Top 5 responses and create our Starter Kits from that information.

We then priced and compared to store-bought products. Each section has a comparison for your information, but remember these are just general prices. You should take into account that some things are cheaper, more expensive or different in different places around the world.

If the kit doesn't suit you, create your own. This is what's so good about making your own products: you are the boss; you decide what's best for you.

THE COST BENEFITS OF USING ESSENTIAL OILS

The main benefit of using Essential Oils when making your own products is that a little goes a long way.

Usually you can buy your Essential Oils in 17 ml, 15 ml, 12 ml or 6 ml Bottles. For every 1 milliliter, you get 20 drops; that means for your 15-ml Bottle, you get 300 drops and for your 12-ml Bottle, you get 240 drops.

With different products ranging from only 10 drops or more, you can see that a little goes a long way.

This is why Essential Oils are a cost-effective way to create your own blends. By simply changing the quantities of Essential Oils, the mix of oils and the base products, you are able to make many products with only a few oils.

I love that I can make up some products I use all the time and then I can just make up enough of a product if I want it for a single use. For example, when my son had warts, I made up a half bottle and applied as per instruction for the two weeks, and I have not needed to use it again.

Similarly I always have on hand air freshener, all-purpose cleanser, antiseptic cream and bath bombs (ideal to throw in the bath with cranky kids).

Sometimes I have many of the Kits made up and sometimes only a few, depending on my needs at that time. I don't have to run down to the shop and then have a product sitting in my cupboard that I may not use again for ages. I'm saving my time and my money.

SECTION 2

The Wonders of Essential Oils

ENJOYING THE BENEFITS OF ESSENTIALS OILS

Essential Oils in their pure state are too highly concentrated to be used directly on the skin, but they provide therapeutic benefits to the body as they are absorbed into the bloodstream via the skin and lungs. The aromatic fragrance has a pleasing and powerful effect on your general well-being.

As the Essential Oils enter the bloodstream, they take their healing powers to the part of the body that is in the most need. When Essential Oils are used around the house, their properties are suitable for surface cleaning and airborne applications.

Because Essential Oils are made from plants and herbs, they give you natural healing properties that are free of any chemicals. They are very concentrated and a little goes a long way. There are over 150 Essential Oils produced, but some are obscure and not readily used.

For your best value in money, quality, and time, we use our ten most popular Essential Oils in all of *The Essential 5* combinations. We also give you information on over twenty more popular Essential Oils.

Used in the right quantities and with other Essential Oils and bases, you can create many different products. Throughout this book you will see again and again the amazing versatility of Essential Oils.

When you start making your own products you not only help yourself, your own body and those of your family but also you help the environment by using natural ingredients.

No chemicals. No chemicals means you're not adding particulates to your home or bodies that could cause a reaction. Chemicals are not good for either you or the environment. Without them, your body will thrive during the cleaning and moisturizing because it will not have to break them down before it starts to get the benefit of the product. Let's face it: the fewer chemicals we use the better it's got to be.

Natural. Without any man-made carcinogens, your body will get a multitude of benefits from the Essential Oils, base products and the synergy of both. You can benefit by adding the healing aromas to your environment while cleaning. By using Essential Oils to sleep, you may reduce the use of store-bought medications.

Simple to make. When you are busy, you don't need more jobs to do; however, you will do things if the benefits outweigh the extra work. By keeping the recipes and process simple, you do reap the benefits. I like the less complicated mixtures and allowing the kids to help is fun and makes one less job for me. If I need a product that I have not previously used, I love that I can make it quickly and use it straightaway.

Fun to make. Kids love it—let them create their own. It's amazing how much more they are willing to clean if they make the product, How much cleaner they will be if they use the soap they helped make!

BUYING ESSENTIAL OILS

When you buy your Essential Oils, remember these simple points to ensure your value for money and quality.

Buy only 100-percent Pure Essential Oils. Check your labels or product information to ensure you get only *100-percent Pure Essential Oil*. This will be stated on the label. You want to use products that have the highest quality and are the most effective.

Shop around. Prices vary considerably from one retailer to the next, so shop around. Try shopping online, but make sure to clarify the products are 100-percent Pure Essential Oil.

Watch the sizes. Don't buy large bottles of Essential Oils at first or unless you know you will use it. Remember that a little goes a long way. Oils in 6 ml to 17 ml Bottles are big enough to start with. By not using them, you add to your expenses.

Follow recipes. With 100-percent pure Essential Oils, you will need a very small amount. More is not necessarily better. If a blend requires four drops of oil, adding eight will not make it better; it will make it stronger—maybe even too strong. (Refer to "Making Your Own Blends") An alteration of the blend may change the properties.

Use the right bottles. Always buy your Essential Oils in blue, amber or dark glass or in aluminum bottles. They need protection from the sunlight that can quickly damage them. Because Essential Oils degrade plastics quickly, always buy 100-percent pure oils (or blends with over a 50-percent Essential Oil ratio) in glass bottles. If oils are supplied in plastic bottles, they will not be 100-percent pure Essential Oils.

WHY QUALITY IS BETTER THAN QUANTITY

To achieve the natural properties of Essential Oils, you need to use 100-percent pure Essential Oils.

NOT Fragrant Oils. Artificially perfumed carrier oils or man-made petroleum based are easy to recognize because the label will say fragrance oil and the cost will be minimal.

NOT Low Grade Oils. Essential Oils in low quality base oils may still be inexpensive but the aroma will not be intense. Usually the bottle will not say 100-percent pure Essential Oil.

NOT "Pure" Oils. Avoid those that have been blended with synthetic oils; these are not natural high quality base oils. This will also be stated on the label either on the front or as part of the ingredients.

Use 100-percent Pure Essential Oils only. Not all 100-percent pure Essential Oils are the same so look closely for those that have 100-percent pure Essential Oil on label, have both the common name and the botanical name (may be written on front of side of bottle), and have droppers inserted in the neck of the bottle (a regulation in most counties because of the strength of Essential Oils). Most bottles will also have warnings of use on the label as well. If buying off the internet, you may find the Essential Oil information on the web site while the bottle has minimal information.

Remember: Quality Not Quantity Is the Secret. Always buy the highest quality available; in the long term, you will save money as they last longer, go farther, and work better.

LOOKING AFTER YOUR OILS

Essential Oils are extremely volatile and can be affected by light, temperature, moisture, air and environment. Look after your Essential Oils and they will last around two years.

Follow a couple of simple rules to get the most from your oils.

- Keep your Essential Oils well sealed. Don't leave the lid off for long periods while you are making products because this can reduce the integrity of the oil.

- Always store 100-percent pure oils (or blends with over 50 percent Essential Oil ratio) in glass bottles, not plastic. Essential Oils degrade plastics quickly.

- Store your Essential Oils in a cool, dry and dark place away from the heat and light. A wooden box is ideal, and some are made especially for Essential Oils.

- Do not store Essential Oils in a refrigerator as it may add moisture and can thicken the oils.

If you look after your Essential Oils and follow these simple recommendations, you will find they will last and you will use up the bottle before the oils expire.

I have a wooden box to keep mine in; it's great for storage and I always know where they are. I put them in top of my linen cupboard out of the way because pure Essential Oils are very concentrated. If you have little children, you should put them up out of reach. These oils can irritate small children in their pure form; see cautions for more information.

THE TOP, THE MIDDLE AND THE BASE OF ESSENTIAL OIL NOTES

All Essential Oils are divided into three note categories:

- Top note
- Middle note
- Base note

These categories can be a little subjective because some Essential Oils are marginal and can claim to be both *top and middle* or *middle and base* notes.

The Essential 5 Oils are all have top and middle notes. Even though a base note would give up more depth, I felt the properties of these 5 versatile Essential Oils were more beneficial than their Aromatic Notes. Where possible you would use a combination of properties and notes

In the Perfume section where using notes is important, I have added two more Essential Oils, Jasmine and Ylang Ylang, to give depth and extra fragrance.

Combining note types when creating blends gives you more character and depth. This is used extensively by manufacturers in cosmetics, body products and perfumery. Today they are also using it in cleaning and household products because they are acknowledging the importance of aromas and how we relate to them.

We have used this knowledge in creating our recipes, and you can too if you decide to create your own.

Top Notes

Top notes are lighter oils which evaporate faster. This is why you will usually detect this oil's aroma first. Top notes are uplifting in scent and usually less expensive in price. Since they are highly volatile and fast acting, they are not very long lasting.

Middle Notes

Middle notes are slightly heavier and tend to last longer than the top notes; they are not usually as noticeable at first and may take a few minutes for their aromas to become obvious. Middle notes are usually warmer and softer than the top notes and may linger for two or three hours

Base Notes

Base notes are the heaviest of all and are the slowest to evaporate. Base notes are used to hold the blend together. These notes may remain for up to 12 hours. The heavier notes tend to be richer and more relaxing and usually are the most expensive of all oils.

TOP NOTES	MIDDLE NOTES	BASE NOTES
denotes Top and Middle note or Middle and Base Note		
Basil	Black Pepper	Cedarwood
Bergamot	Chamomile	Cinnamon *M-B
Citronella	Clary Sage* T-M	Clove
Eucalyptus	Cypress	Frankincense
Grapefruit	Geranium	Ginger
Lemon	Ginger	Myrrh
Lime	Jasmine	Patchouli
Neroli* T-M	Lavender * M-T	Rose
Orange	Marjoram	Sandalwood
Peppermint	Palmarosa	Vetiver
Sage	Petitgrain	Ylang Ylang
Rosemary *T-M	Pine	
	Tree Tea* T-M	
	Thyme	

WHY DIFFERENT OILS HAVE DIFFERENT PRICES

Huge volumes are needed to produce a single kilo of pure Essential Oil. For example, a kilo requires approximately

- 200 kg of fresh Lavender flowers or
- 2,000-3,000 kg of Rose petals or
- 3,000 Lemons

As you can see, there is a large difference in the quantity of raw materials needed to create the Essential Oils. This along with availability of the raw material will be reflected in the prices. If the products you are buying cost the same, then check the quality; prices can vary considerably.

For this reason the price of oils depends on the plant from which they are extracted. Rose and Sandalwood oils, for example, are more expensive than Lavender and Lemon.

Some oils are so expensive and concentrated that they are mixed in jojoba oil at 3 percent or 6 percent to make them available for general purchase. Use these just like 100-percent pure oils since the strength will still be suitable. You may find Chamomile, Rose and Jasmine among others blended like this.

CAUTIONS USING ESSENTIAL OILS

- Essential Oils must not be taken internally.
- Always purchase oils in tamper-proof lids because 100-percent oils are very concentrated.
- Do not exceed the recommended ratios.
- Keep away from eyes. Wash immediately with warm water. If burning occurs, seek medical advice.
- Remember to spot test on a small area of healthy skin for any topical applications to ensure there is no reaction. Always dilute oil for spot test into recipe blend or mix one drop of Essential Oils to five drops of Base Oil for body applications such as common ailments, massage, skin care, and hair care.
- Always use pure Essential Oils diluted (exception Lavender and Tree may be used neat).
- For those with extremely sensitive skin or allergic skin, do a patch test on any oil before using. You may need to avoid Basil, Bergamot, Thyme and Tea Tree.
- If you have high blood pressure, avoid Eucalyptus, Rosemary, Thyme
- If you have low blood pressure, avoid Ylang Ylang, Marjoram and large quantities of Lavender.
- Epileptics should avoid Basil, Sage, Rosemary and Eucalyptus,
- Pregnant women should avoid all oils (for massage) in the first three months; instead, they should use Base Oil only. Oils that are considered safe are Lavender, Chamomile, Grapefruit, Ylang Yang, Geranium, Orange, Cypress, Rosemary, Frankincense, Peppermint, Ginger and Bergamot.
- Children can use a blend at half the strength recommended for adults. Ideal Essential Oils are Lavender and Chamomile.
- If the skin is exposed to strong sunlight, avoid using citrus oils on skin. These include Bergamot, Lemon, and Orange.

SECTION 3

Bases - Bringing It All Together

Understanding the Need for Base Oils and Base Products

Since pure Essential Oils are very concentrated, they will need to be diluted in a base oil or product for use. Without base oils or products, Essential Oils may be harmful and irritate your skin (with the exception of Lavender and Tea Tree—refer to "A-Z Essential Oils" for more information) or cause damage to surfaces.

BASE OILS

Base oils help Essential Oils penetrate the skin and enable the body to absorb the properties of the Essential Oils.

These are especially important when using Essential Oils for massage or topical application. Use high quality cold pressed oil that has maintained its vitamin and mineral content and has better absorption ability than cheaper, processed oils.

Base oils are vegetable oils used either by themselves or in conjunction with Essential Oils to give you a product that can be applied directly onto the skin for massage and used for spot applications or any body application.

There are lots of different oils—Safflower, Apricot, Avocado, Olive Oil, Sunflower, Evening Primrose, Grape seed, Hazelnut, Jojoba, Macadamia, Rosehip, Sweet Almond, Wheat Germ, Peanut to name a few. Listed below are some of these base oils and their properties and uses.

COMMONLY USE BASE OILS AND THEIR PROPERTIES

Apricot Kernel Oil

Color: slight yellow
Apricot Kernel oil is nutritious for the skin, especially aging or sun damaged skin, but is suitable for all skin types. It is rich in vitamin A, has very little scent, and absorbs quickly into the skin.

Avocado Oil

Color: dark green
Avocado oil contains protein, vitamin, fatty acids and lecithin. Use it in a dilution of 10 percent. It is good for all skin types, for eczema and for dry and dehydrated skins.

Evening Primrose

Color: medium yellow
Excellent for skin conditions such as stretch marks, Evening Primrose oil also assists with reducing water retention. It should be used with other carrier oils as 10 percent of the total blend because it will leave an oily residue on skin. Evening Primrose has high levels of essential fatty acids and soothes inflammations, It is useful with dandruff applications.

Grapeseed Oil

Color: very pale green or almost clear
Grapeseed oil is a general all-around oil useful for massages and all skin types; it contains minerals, vitamins and proteins.

Jojoba Oil

Color: yellow
Not really oil, Jojoba oil is actually a wax; it has a balancing effect on skin. Because it is highly penetrative, it should be used with other carrier oils as 10 percent of blend. It is rich in Vitamin E and will not turn rancid like other oils because it has antioxidant properties. It is beneficial for body, face and hair treatments. Use Jojoba oil with expensive Essential Oils to make the oil less expensive. Because it is a wax, it does reduce the clarity of Essential Oils and is usually in a 3-percent blend.

Olive Oil

Color: yellow or slightly green
Olive oil is not only used for skin and hair applications, it is also used extensively in cooking. It is a soothing oil, suitable for hair care and cosmetics.

Sunflower Oil

Color: light yellow
One of the most common and well known oils, Sunflower oil is suitable for all skin types and contains both vitamins and minerals. This oil can be used for most areas of aromatherapy.

Safflower Oil

Color: light yellow
Safflower oil is popular in massage blends because it is easily absorbed and can be washed from sheets without heavy staining. It is rich in linolenic acid (Omega-6) and low in viscosity making it suitable for skin and hair conditioning products. It is odorless.

Sweet Almond Oil

Color: golden yellow
Sweet Almond oil is rich in proteins, polyunsaturates and vitamin D. It is a light versatile oil suitable for all skin types and is considered extremely nourishing. It has little scent and is popular for massage therapists. Sweet Almond absorbs into skin at an average speed, feeling slightly oily.

Wheat Germ Oil

Color: yellowish orange
Wheat Germ oil is a very strong oil suitable for prematurely aging skin, eczema and psoriasis. It should be used as 10 percent of the total blend of oil.

COMMON USE BASE PRODUCTS AND THEIR PROPERTIES

BASE PRODUCTS

Base products combined with Essential Oils for household cleaning and gifts have been around for centuries with records showing uses as far back as ancient Roman times and in Egypt, Greece and India.

Base products range from everyday common products such as Bicarb (Bicarbonate soda), soaps, salt, vinegar, Vitamin V creams, Aloe Vera, and eggs along with many other commonly used ingredients.

Understanding that base oils and products have their own properties (attribute, characteristic or ability) enables you to expand the range of recipes and products you may create.

Aloe Vera Gel

Aloe Vera Gel has many properties. It is an antibiotic and an astringent that can inhibit pain, stimulate cell growth, and inhibit scar tissue. It assists in rejuvenating the skin and contains B12, protein, amino acids, and enzymes. It is renowned for its usefulness on burns, sunburn and dry skin.

Base Cream

Sorebolene Cream, Vitamin E Cream, or Organic Body Cream

Sorbolene cream is a gentle but effective cream made of 10 percent glycerin. A good quality cream is made to a dermatological standard and is suitable for most people. (If an allergic reaction occurs, cease use and try a different product.) A natural Vitamin E cream or an organic natural body cream is also suitable as a base. Make sure your cream is thick because adding the Essential Oils will thin out the cream; a thicker cream product is much better. Remember: because of the thickness and richness of this cream, a little will go a long way.

Base Oil

A good quality cold press carrier oil is essential for use in hair care recipes. There are several you can use (refer to section on Base Oils for more detailed information). I use Sweet Almond oil, Olive oil and Safflower oil. Sweet Almond and Olive oils can be purchased at supermarkets or health food stores. Safflower and other oils can be purchased from health shops. The quantities are the same for any base oil, so in the recipes that call for base oil, use the one you like, or is in your price range, or is the easiest to get. The base oil in hair care products allows you to blend the Essential Oils and penetrate the hair follicles.

Bicarb (*Sodium Bicarbonate* or Baking Soda)

Bicarb is a natural substance made from sodium Bicarbonate and sodium carbonate. Also called baking soda, it is not to be confused with baking powder which is usually found in smaller containers and has none of Bicarb's benefits. It's great for cleaning, deodorizing, softening water, and air freshening. It's also good for polishing surfaces, fish tanks, and windows.

Detergent or Pure Soap

Try to get a bio-degradable, non-scented, natural, and environmentally friendly blend of detergent or pure soap. Depending on your preference, you can use a simple detergent or pure soap since both have properties that cut through dirt and grease. Use a dishwashing liquid for home-made recipes or use pure soap (such as Sunlight, Castle or Lux). Grate the soap and add to water.

Eggs

Eggs are a great component in hair care products. They contain natural fatty acid that restore the hair's natural shine and assist with reducing split ends. Eggs can be combined with other products to help combat frizz and restore shine to dry and dull hair.

Epsom Salts (*Magnesium Sulfate Heptahydrate*)

Epsom Salts is used for softening skin and relaxing sore muscles. They help raise the body's serotonin levels which help elevate your mood, improve sleep and concentration, and reduce stress. Combining this with the appropriate Essential Oil gives you a wonderful product. Soaking in a bath with *Epsom Salts* is not only enjoyable but is very good for your body and your mind.

Pure Soap (Liquid Soap Mix)

A great pure soap is the basis for many products. Use a pure gentle soap, such as Sunlight, Castle or Lux.

Liquid Soap Mix

Grate a half bar of soap and add to 500 ml Water. Place broken up soap (or grated) into a saucepan or microwave-proof dish with water and bring to boil. Boil until the soap has become a slurry; this should take approximately 10-15 minutes. Allow to cool until just warm and pour into blender. (Do not put hot ingredients into blender.) Blend until smooth and pour into a bottle. Store and use for all recipes requiring soap.

Salt

Salt is a natural abrasive product, but remember to use it gently on softer surfaces. Do not use it on stainless steel surfaces as it will scratch. Salt is ideal if you need a harsher abrasive than Bicarb. It is great on built-up grime in ovens, on baking trays, and on saucepans.

Vinegar

Vinegar is a multipurpose liquid created from the fermentation of ethanol; the key ingredient is acetic acid which gives it the acidic taste. Vinegar cuts through grease and works as a mild disinfectant and deodorizer. It inhibits bacteria and mildew and it is fabulous for wooden floors.

Vodka

To make perfumes and astringents, you need a alcohol base. As pure alcohol is very expensive and hard to find, vodka is suitable. You may use brandy or another alcohol but be aware that their aromas will become part of the blend.

HOW TO MIX AND USE ESSENTIAL OILS WITH BASES

When making your own blends, be sure you use clean bottles. If you are recycling old bottles, give them a thorough cleaning.

When making products for first aid, skin care, perfumes, or other high concentrated uses, make sure you use dark *glass* bottles to mix and store your oils. Higher concentrations of Essential Oils absorb into plastic and break down the structure.

For lower concentrated blends in products for household cleaning, hair care, sleeping, some gifts, relaxation massage, and bath products, using plastic bottles, jars, and spray bottles is fine. To prolong shelf life, always store your Essential Oils, base oils, and home-made products away from the sun.

In the following sections, you'll find all the information you will need to blend with confidence.

- ✓ So You Want to Make Your Own Products
- ✓ Effective Applications—Using Your Products
- ✓ Bottles and Jars: What's Best and How to Recycle
- ✓ Creating Labels: Without Them, You Would Be Lost

SECTION 4

Making Your Own

So You Want To Make Your Own Products

Making your own products is as simple as following a basic cooking recipe (without the cooking). Just add the products per the instructions and, *voilà, **you have your own product**!*

To make products for body applications, first add in your base oil and then add Essential Oil drops. To blend, tip the bottle upside down several times and then roll the bottle around in your palm to disperse the Essential Oil through the base oil.

When making products for surface, airborne, and other applications, follow the recipe instructions.

Below is a general ratio (percentage Essential Oil to base product) guideline. Sometimes I have adjusted the ratio for a specific situation.

Body Application 1:1
1 drop of Essential Oil to 1 ml of Base Oil or Cream

Body Massage 1:2
1 drop of Essential Oil to 2 ml of Base Oil

Air Spray 1:10
1 drop of Essential Oil to 10 ml Base Product

Inhalations 1:100
1 drop of Essential Oil to 100 ml Water

Skin Care 1:1
1 drop Essential Oil to 1 ml Base Product

Hair Care 1:2
1 drop Essential Oil to 2 ml Base Product

Effective Applications — Using your Products

There are many ways to use Essential Oils and benefit from the properties and aromas. These can be beneficial to almost everyone. In this chapter, you will find how to use Essential Oil-based products from the well known methods such as massage to bathing, natural blends, oil burners and inhalations.

Aromatherapy works to promote relaxation and mood enhancement through the nervous system and can be a wonderful benefit to your body, mind, and spirit.

The properties of Essential Oil help with body complaints, cleaning, sleeping, and stress; they leave you feeling uplifted or relaxed depending on the Essential Oils you use.

Here are some of the ways to use Essential Oils.

Atomizers
Always use glass bottles with a ratio of 1 drop Essential Oil to 5 ml distilled water. This is ideal for face spray.

Bathing
Add 6-10 drops of Essential Oils to a full bath. Agitate the water to disperse the Essential Oil evenly before entering the water. Use warm water to relax; use hot water to revitalize. Drop into base of shower after washing and, upon rinsing body, inhale and enjoy the beneficial aromas.

Blend
Use a ratio of 1 drop Essential Oil to 1 ml Base Oil. Use may be diluted to 1:2 for body massage oil.

Bottles and Jars

Create your own products, creating common ailment products. Use a ratio of 1 drop Essential Oil to 1 ml base product. For cleaning and other application, see relevant sections.

Compress

Disperse Essential Oils (may be pre-blended with Base Oil) into approximately 250 ml of water. Stir the water thoroughly to disperse the Essential Oil. Place a cloth or gauze into the water, squeeze out, and place onto the affected area. Use a cold compress for headaches, migraines, aching eyes, or tension and for ankles on long flights. Leave the compress in place for approximately 20 minutes or until it gets warm. Hot compresses may be used for boils and as part of injury treatment.

Direct Application

With the exception of Lavender and Tee Tree, direction application is not generally recommended (unless on the advice of a qualified practitioner).

Footbath

Disperse 6 drops of Essential Oil into large bowl of warm-to-hot water (or directly into foot spa). Stir the water. In the bottom of a bowl, place large rounded stones or marbles and roll the soles of your feet around on them. (In a foot spa, turn on and enjoy. Use the heat and massage setting for the ultimate pleasure.) Soak for a minimum of 15 minutes.

Humidifiers

Add Essential Oils to the water and follow the humidifier's instructions.

Inhalation

Add 5-10 drops of Essential Oil to a large bowl of boiling water. Stir quickly with a metal spoon (wooden spoon will absorb the oils). Place face over bowl and inhale. For a more intense inhalation, place a towel over your head and bowl and inhale gently. This application is an invaluable aid for relief of colds, sinuses, and headaches. It is also ideal to hydrate and cleanse skin and improve stamina. For a quick inhalation, add 2 drops of Essential Oil neat—not diluted—to a handkerchief or tissue and inhale.

Massage

Massage is one of the oldest forms of treatment. Use a ratio of 1 drop Essential Oil to 2 ml of Base Oil. An aromatic massage is a wonderful experience and will leave you feeling wonderful for days.

Oils Burners and Diffusers

Made especially to use with Essential Oils, oil burners and diffusers warm the oil and release the molecules into the atmosphere. When purchasing an oil burner, look for one with a large top bowl. Fill the top bowl with warm water and add 10 drops of Essential Oil. Place a tea light candle in the bottom section and light. The Essential Oil will gently fragrance the air and, depending on the properties of the oil, either create an aromatic ambience or rid the air of insects, bad smells, bad moods and the like. Use the diffuser per the recommended instructions

Shower

Wash as usual and place a couple of drops of your favorite blend on your sprayer and rub over your body as you stand under the running water. Breathe deeply and inhale the aromatic steam.

BOTTLES AND JARS: WHAT'S BEST

You can purchase your bottles and jars from specialty suppliers or supermarkets (small selection), or you can recycle old bottles and jars from around the house.

Ensure that the bottle or jar is very clean. After cleaning, boil all glass containers to make them sterile; steam clean plastic containers.

For higher concentrated products (ratios 1:1), use glass bottles or jars. For all other products, plastic bottles and jars are suitable.

Boiling. Place bottles and jars in large saucepan on stove. Fill with water and slowly bring to the boil. Boil for 5-10 minutes. Turn off the stove and remove bottles very carefully. There will be hot water around the bottle and inside the bottle.

Steaming. Place bottles and jars in a steamer and boil water underneath for at least 5-10 minutes. Leave in steamer until cooled.

Sterilizers. Use baby sterilizers for both glass and plastic bottles.

CREATING LABELS: WITHOUT THEM, YOU WOULD BE LOST

Start creating. Remember to label your products for easy use

Label example

Air Freshener - Kitchen
2 teaspoon Bicarb, 1/4 cup white Vinegar and water,
Lavender 4 drops, Lemon 4 drops, Tea Tree 2 drops
SHAKE WELL BEFORE USE

Or simply

Air Freshener

SECTION 5

House Cleaning Naturally

Some people enjoy cleaning, some people love cleaning, some tolerate it and some do it because "it has to be done." I'm somewhere between tolerate and "has to be done"—definitely not in the love area. Put on some music, grab the kids, grab my great products, and I get it done.

I want products that work; I don't want to have to repeat. So if I can have effective products that are natural and chemical free and smell divine, then that's a bonus!

I always have my Top 10 House Cleaning Kit products premixed and in a cleaning bucket ready for use, but for most of the other products, I quickly blend them if I need them.

With recipes that are even simpler that the original ones I have been using over the years, I can have products on hand quickly and easily. The kids are now mixing them for me. They love the fizzing of Bicarb and Vinegar. They love the fragrances and the way the products are created. (If only I could get them as enthusiastic about cleaning their rooms!)

I find that an added benefit to using Essential Oils is the aroma works on your senses while you clean. You get the calm benefit of Lavender, the uplifting aroma of Lemon, and the refreshing and invigorating fragrances of Tea Tree and Eucalyptus (especially great when colds and flu are around).

With the use of natural products and 5 Essential Oils, you can create a complete home cleaning system that is less expensive than buying individual cleaning products.

HOW TO BENEFIT AT HOME

This section has been written to give you clear, simple, and effective solutions for household cleaning. If you are a first-time user of Essential Oils for cleaning, you will find the instruction clear and easy to follow. If you already use Essential Oils for cleaning, you can add these recipes to your knowledge and create your own blends using the ratio information provided with each recipe.

The ratio tells you how much Essential Oil to Vinegar, Bicarb, water or other element to use. This allows you to add your own Essential Oil creations from the hundreds of Essential Oils available.

For many years I have used Essential Oils for first aid and relaxation, but I truly got my money's worth when I started using them around the house. My cleaning bill went down. Cleaning didn't become any harder by using the natural products, and I knew I was helping my family's health and wellbeing by using fewer chemicals around the house.

By using the Essential Oil properties, I was about to create blends that were germ busting and antiseptic. I could use aromas that smelled great and created a clean environment. I love that if I discovered I needed a product while I was cleaning, I didn't need to go to the shop to get it; I could make it straightaway and use it. I did not have to put that job off to another day (it does have to get done).

THE COST COMPARISON OF YOUR HOUSEHOLD CLEANING STARTER KIT

When you first purchase high quality, 100-percent pure Essential Oils, you may think that you have spent a lot of money for such a small quality of oils, but a little goes a long way.

Essential Oils from a 12 ml bottle will provide you with 240 drops of Essential Oil. Compare the cost of buying the ten products.

Purchased Products (Generic or Cheapest Product Available)	Cost	Products Created Using Essential 5 Essential Oils and Household Products	Cost
Air Freshener–125 ml	$2.00	Air Freshener–125 ml	$0.35
All-Purpose Cleanser–500 ml	$6.00	All-Purpose Cleanser–500 ml	$1.20
Baking Soda–500 g	$1.00	Baking Soda–500 g	$1.00
Disinfectant–2 liters	$2.40	Disinfectant–2 liters	$1.20
Dishwashing Liquid–500 ml	$3.30	Dishwashing Liquid–500 ml	$3.30
Floor Cleaner–750 ml	$2.30	Floor Cleaner–750 ml	$0.40
Insect Repellent–300 ml	$2.80	Insect Repellent–300 ml	$0.50
Glass Cleaner–500 ml	$3.20	Glass Cleaner–500 ml	$0.65
Surface Cleaner Spray–500 ml	$4.40	Surface Cleaner Spray–500 ml	$1.05
Vinegar–1 liter	$1.00	Vinegar–1 liter	$1.00
TOTAL COST	**$28.40**	**TOTAL COST**	**$10.65**

Plus, the Essential 5 products are multi-usable, and some of the products have other uses.

- **Air Freshener.** Use as a room deodorizer, ironing aid, or curtain freshener.

- **All-Purpose Cleanser.** Use in any room in the house that needs an abrasive cleaner; use for ovens, showers, fridges, air conditioners, bathrooms, benches, cups, drawers, and microwaves

- **Baking Soda Shaker.** Use as a general all-purpose abrasive. Use to clean stainless steel or to prevent odor in shoes.

- **Disinfectant.** Use to eliminate harmful bugs or clean children's rooms.

- **Dishwashing Liquid.** Use to wash dishes, floors, and stairs.

- **Floor Cleaner.** Use on tile, vinyl, or wood floors (test first!).

- **Insect Repellent.** Use as a spray or in an oil burner.

- **Mirror and Glass Cleaner.** Use on mirrors, windows, glass, eye glasses, and car windows.

- **Surface Spray.** Use for a quick wipe to clean fridges, showers, basins, vanity, benches, walls, and other surfaces.

- **Vinegar Spray.** Use as antibacterial surface cleaner, polish car chrome, spray car windows to keep them frost free, and clean eye glasses. It is a must-have for jellyfish and blue bottle stings. It removes fruit stains and onion smells from hands.

RECIPES: HOUSEHOLD CLEANING STARTER KIT

Ingredients List

Your will need the following items to create one complete Starter Kit

- ✓ Lavender Essential Oil
- ✓ Lemon Essential Oil
- ✓ Tea Tree Essential Oil
- ✓ Eucalyptus Essential Oil
- ✓ 6 250-ml Clean Spray Bottles, New Or Recycled
- ✓ 2 250-ml Clean Bottles (Squirt or Pour), New or Recycled
- ✓ 1 Clean Large Salt Shaker, or Jar with Holes In Lid
- ✓ 280 grams Bicarb Soda
- ✓ 690 ml Vinegar
- ✓ 300 ml Liquid Soap or Washing Up Liquid
- ✓ 150 ml Vegetable Oil

1. AIR FRESHENER SPRAY

Ratio: 15 drops Essential Oil : 250 ml Water

250 ml Spray Bottle
15 drops Essential Oils as below (Blend Suggestions)
250 ml Boiled (Cooled) Water

To freshen and deodorize your house, don't mask the bad smells; eliminate them. With any of the below blends, you can create a great air freshener, using Essential Oils to suit your needs.

Mix 1: Add 10 drops of Essential Oils into a bottle of water and shake well. Shake before each use.

Blend Suggestions:
- Welcoming. Welcome people into your home. This invokes memories of peace in most people.
  Lavender 15 drops
- All-purpose. A blend suitable for every room, this freshens the air and contains bacterial properties.
  Lavender 8 drops, Lemon 4 drops, Eucalyptus 3 drops
- Bloom. Ideal for eliminating cooking odor in the kitchen.
  Lavender 6 drops, Lemon 5 drops, Tea Tree 4 drops
- Smell Ease. Remove the unpleasant odor associated with bathrooms and laundries.
  Lemon 10 drops, Eucalyptus 3 drops, Lavender 2 drops

Other Uses:
- Ironing aid. Spray directly onto clothes and then iron.
- Room deodorizer. Eliminate stale and unpleasant smells.
- Curtain freshener. Spray directly onto curtains and allow the warm of the sun to intensify the beautiful natural Essential Oil aromas.

2. BICARB SHAKER

Ratio: Bicarb only

Large Salt Shaker
Bicarb

Use a large salt shaker, talc powder bottle, or container (jar) with holes pierced into lid. If Bicarb is needed as an abrasive, use it alone. For added removal of built-up grime, use it as a Surface Spray or All-Purpose Cleanser. Bicarb is easier and more practical in the shaker than pouring it out of a box. You seem to use less when the powder is evenly distributed.

Other Uses:
- Kids. Kids will love using this. Shake onto surface, spray with Vinegar, and watch it fizz. Let the kids wipe the counter and enjoy the fizzing feeling on their fingers. This is cleaning done with fun!!!
- Stainless Steel. Cleans and removes minor rust stains.
- Odor eliminator. Use on shoes, carpets, and pet areas.

3. ALL-PURPOSE CLEANSER

Ratio: 20 drops Essential Oil : 60 ml Vinegar : 50 ml Soap : 140 ml Water

Mix1:
250 ml Sauce (Squirt) Bottle
140 ml Boiled (Warm) Water
60 ml Vinegar
50 ml Soap or Washing Liquid
2 tablespoons Bicarb
10 drops Lemon Essential Oil
5 drops Eucalyptus Essential Oil
3 drops Lavender Essential Oil
2 drops Tea Tree Essential Oil

This recipe makes a wonderful all-purpose cleanser you can use throughout the household. It is heavier than a surface spray with a gentle abrasive quality and soap for removal of grease build up. This cleaner is antibacterial and a disinfectant.

Mix: Mix this in a glass bowl or jug; cool and pour into a bottle. Pour in ½ of warm water and add Bicarb; stir until dissolved. Add to this mixture ½ of the Vinegar and allow the mixture to rinse and lower; then add the rest of the Vinegar. Add liquid soap and stir until blended. Add Essential Oils and pour in remaining warm water. Stir well and cool before using.

Other Uses:
- Benches. Clean any surface with this gentle abrasive cleaner.
- Fridges. Use for fresh odor and sparkling clean look.
- Showers and bathrooms. Helps eliminate build up.
- Coffee cups. Remove coffee stains.
- Drawers. Remove grime and marks.
- Microwaves. Clean inside and out.

4. DISINFECTANT

Ratio: 20 drops Essential Oil : 70 ml Vinegar : 180 ml Water

250 ml Spray Bottle
70 ml Vinegar
180 ml Boiled (Cooled) *Water*
10 drops Lavender Essential Oil
6 drops Lemon Essential Oil
4 drops Eucalyptus Essential Oil

Create an effective disinfectant to use around the house and spray onto most surfaces. Wipe dry or leave it moist behind toilets, fridges, washing machines, backs of cupboards, and along skirting boards—anywhere germs may harbor.

Mix: Mix in a glass bowl or jug; cool and pour into a spray bottle. Combine Vinegar with Bicarb (be sure to allow for the rising and foaming of Vinegar and Bicarb). Add Water and Essential Oils. Shake well.

5. DISHWASHING LIQUID

Ratio: 10 drops Essential Oil : 250 ml Dishwashing Liquid

Dishwashing Liquid, Natural, Biodegradable
or Make your own (See Below Recipe)
10 drops Essential Oil blend as below (Blend Suggestions)

Adding Essential Oils to your natural dishwashing liquid will give you a product that not only works as well as before but now has the additional benefits of the Essential Oils. Quick and simple, add this mixture to your bottle of dishwashing liquid or add 3 drops to your sink every time you wash up.

Mix: Add 12 drops of Essential Oil from the below blends to your biodegradable, natural dishwashing liquid (250 ml Bottle).

Make Your Own Natural Dishwashing Liquid

500 ml Sauce Bottle
5 tablespoons Soap Flakes or Soap (grated) – Castle, Sunlight or Lux soaps
450 ml Boiled (Warm) Water
2 tablespoons Vinegar
2 teaspoons Glycerin
12 drops of Essential Oils from blends above

Mix together soap and water until soap is dissolved. Add glycerin, Vinegar, and essential oils. Shake well. This recipe will clean well, but will not foam, create bubbles, or change water color. (You will get used to this.)

6. FLOOR CLEANER

Ratio: 10 drops Essential Oils : Bucket of Hot Water

Mop
Bucket
Dishwashing Detergent or Soap Flakes (or Soap Grated)
10 drops of Essential Oils as below (Blend Suggestions)

Mop the floors with a clean damp mop using one of the following blends. No need to rinse. You can use the dishwashing liquid blend instead of creating a new mix.

Mix: Add 10 drops of Essential Oils into a bucket of warm water with detergent or soap. You can premix the blends into another 12 ml Glass Bottle or simple drop directly into the bucket from the original bottles.

Blend Suggestions:
- Welcoming. Lavender 10 drops
- Bacterial. Lavender 5 drops, Lemon 3 drops, Eucalyptus 2 drops
- Kitchen. Lavender 4 drops, Lemon 4 drops, Tea Tree 2 drops
- Bathroom. Lemon 5 drops, Eucalyptus 3 drops, Lavender 2 drops.

7. INSECT REPELLENT

Ratio of Mix 1 and 2: 20 drops Essential Oil : 100 ml Water : 150 ml Vegetable Oil

Mix 1
250 ml Spray Bottle
100 ml Water
8 drops Lavender Essential Oil
5 drops Tea Tree Essential Oil
2 drops Eucalyptus Essential Oil
150 ml Vegetable Oil (or any oil, such as olive, sunflower, etc.)

Mix 2
Remove 3 drops Lavender
Add 3 drops Citronella Essential Oil (not part of Essential 4 oils)
Follow recipe as above.

A natural insect repellent is good for all the family. As many insect repellents contain DEET, a harsh chemical that can cause skin and body reactions, this is an ideal solution to alleviate the use of a very harsh chemical. This blend may be used as a house spray; spray it around windows, directly into the air and behind fridges—wherever creepy crawlies hide.

For oil burners, use a blend of Essential Oils without water or Base Oil. This is ideal to reduce mosquitoes and flies in rooms.

Mix: Mix the water and Base Oil together and add Essential Oils. Shake well. This product will need to be shaken before each use as no dispersant was added. (A dispersant is a chemical to stop the ingredients from separating. A quick shake does the same thing.)

8. MIRRORS and WINDOWS

Ratio: 10 Essential Oil : 250 ml Vinegar

250 ml Spray Bottle
250 ml Vinegar
10 drops Lemon Essential Oil

Mirrors and windows shine up beautifully when cleaned and then wiped dry with newspaper (environmentally friendly and lint free).

Mix: In a spray bottle, blend water with 250 ml Vinegar and Essential Oil. Shake well.

Spray on mirrors and wipe with damp cloth or newspaper; then wipe dry with newspaper.

9. SURFACE SPRAY

Ratio: 15 drops Essential Oil: 60 ml Vinegar: 2 teaspoons Bicarb : 190 ml Water

250 ml Spray Bottle
2 teaspoons Bicarb
60 ml Vinegar
190 ml Boiled (Warm) Water
15 drops of Essential Oils as below (Blend Suggestions)

This surface spray is great for quick wipe downs when an abrasive isn't needed. Use it on counter tops and any surface that needs cleaning using antibacterial cleaning agents without chemicals

Blend Suggestions:
- Germ Busting. Use wherever germs and bugs harbor.
  Lemon 9 drops, Eucalyptus 4 drops, Lavender 2 drops
- Aromatic. Welcoming and relaxing; ideal for bedrooms.
  Lavender 8 drops, Lemon 4 drops, Eucalyptus 3 drops

Mix: Add Bicarb, and then slowly add in Vinegar (to allow for rising and foaming of Vinegar and Bicarb). Mix together and fill with water. Shake well. Add Essential Oils from blends above and shake again. Always shake before use as no dispersant was added to keep the ingredients together (usually chemical-based additive). A quick shake will do the same thing.

Other Uses:
- Fridges, inside and out.
- Bathrooms, for the shower, vanity, basins, and tiles.
- Kitchens, for sinks, benches, walls, and quick wipe downs.
- Lounge Rooms and Family Rooms, for shelving and walls.

10. VINEGAR SPRAY

Ratio: 250 ml Vinegar

250 ml Spray Bottle
250 ml Vinegar

A pure blend of Vinegar can be used by itself or as part of a cleaning system. This spray is ideal by itself for cleaning mirrors, glass and windows and with Bicarb for cleaning.

Other Uses:
- Polish car chrome.
- Spray car windows to keep them frost free.
- Clean eye glasses.
- Use as a must-have for jellyfish and blue bottle stings.
- Remove fruit stains and onion smell from hands.

Did you know?

Essential Oils have been used in cleaning for centuries. The Romans use Essential Oils to fumigate their temples. Hippocrates fumigated an entire Greek city with Essential Oils to prevent the spread of diseases.

For centuries most monasteries and convents in Europe planted and used herbs and Essential Oils in everyday life for cleaning and herbal remedies.

RECIPES: A-Z OF HOUSEHOLD CLEANING PRODUCT

AIR FRESHENER SPRAY

Ratio: 15 drops Essential Oil : 250 ml Water

250 ml Spray Bottle
15 drops Essential Oils as below (Blend Suggestions)
250 ml Boiled (Cooled) Water

To freshen and deodorize your house, don't mask the bad smells; eliminate them. With any of the below blends, you can create a great air freshener, using Essential Oils to suit your needs.

Mix: 10 drops of Essential Oils into a bottle of water and shake well. Shake before each use.

Blend Suggestions:
- Welcoming. Lavender 15 drops
- All-purpose. Lavender 8 drops, Lemon 4 drops, Eucalyptus 3 drops
- Bloom. Lavender 6 drops, Lemon 5 drops, Tea Tree 4 drops
- Smell Ease. Lemon 10 drops, Eucalyptus 3 drops, Lavender 2 drops

ALL-PURPOSE CLEANSER

Ratio: 20 drops Essential Oil : 60 ml Vinegar : 50 ml Soap : 140 ml Water

Mix 1:
250 ml Sauce (Squirt) Bottle
140 ml Boiled (Warm) Water
60 ml Vinegar
50 ml Soap or Washing Liquid
2 tablespoons Bicarb
10 drops Lemon Essential Oil
5 drops Eucalyptus Essential Oil
3 drops Lavender Essential Oil
2 drops Tea Tree Essential Oil

This recipe makes a wonderful all-purpose cleanser you can use throughout the household. It is heavier than a surface spray with a gentle abrasive quality and soap for removal of grease build up. This cleaner is antibacterial and a disinfectant.

Mix: Mix this in a glass bowl or jug; cool and pour into a bottle.
Pour in ½ of warm water and add Bicarb; stir until dissolved.
Add to this mixture ½ of the Vinegar and allow the mixture to rinse and lower; then add the rest of the Vinegar. Add liquid soap and stir until blended. Add Essential Oils and pour in remaining warm water. Stir well and cool before using.

ANTS

250 ml Spray Bottle
40 ml Vinegar
250 ml Water
10 drops Eucalyptus Essential Oil (Use Peppermint Essential Oil as replacement)
10 drops Lemon Essential Oil

Discourage ants by making up a solution to spray along any point of entry such as a window sill or door. You can also drop it directly onto window ledges or cotton wool or drop it on a cloth and wipe over ledges.

Mix: Combine Essential Oils with Vinegar and fill bottle with water. Shake Well. Essential Oils are great to inhibit ants from entering the house; drop onto window ledges and door frames.

AIR CONDITIONERS
All-Purpose Cleanser

It is important to clean the air conditioner and its filters regularly. Wipe the outside of air conditioner with the All-Purpose Cleanser.

AIR CONDITIONER FILTERS
Air Freshener Spray

Wash under tap and clean of all dirt and grime. Wipe dry or shake dry and spray with Air Freshener Spray this will give the fresh aromatic fragrance when the air conditioner is turned on. You can make this blend any of the Air Freshener blends; the Bacterial Blend is great for winter to assist in the elimination of airborne particles of germs of colds and flu.

BICARB SHAKER

Use this shaker when you need to use Bicarb as an abrasive. Bicarb is easier and more practical in the shaker than pouring it out of a box. You seem to use less since the powder is evenly distributed.

BATHROOMS
Germ Busting Spray

250 ml Spray Bottle
2 teaspoon Bicarb
50 ml Vinegar
200 ml Boiled (Warm) Water
5 drops Lemon Essential Oil
3 drops Eucalyptus Essential Oil
2 drops Lavender Essential Oil

or All-Purpose Cleanser

The bathroom harbors many germs and bugs. Unless appropriate cleaning methods are used, it can be a place where germs thrive and multiply.

Mix: Mix Vinegar and Bicarb (to allow for rising and foaming of Vinegar and Bicarb). Fill with Water and shake well. Then add 10 drops of Essential Oils and shake again. Shake before use.

Grime Cleaner
Bicarb Shaker, Germ Buster Spray, or All-Purpose Cleanser

Mix: Sprinkle Bicarb over surfaces and, using damp cloth, clean all surfaces. This creates an abrasive cleaner for cleaning away grime. Then spray the area with full strength Germ Busting Spray. Rinse thoroughly and wipe over with dry cloth.

BENCHES

500 ml Spray Bottle
20 drops Essential Oils as below

Mix 1: *500 ml Boiled (Warm) Water*

Mix 2: *500 ml Boiled (Warm) Water*
250 ml Vinegar

Mix 1: *Tea Tree 10 drops, Lemon 10 drops, and Water*

Mix 2: *Tea Tree 10 drops, Lemon 10 drops water, Vinegar or All-Purpose Cleanser or Air Freshener Spray*

Tea tree oil can be used with lemon in spray bottle to wipe down benches; this mixture will hinder the growth of fungus and mildew. Always patch test before using on surface.

Mix 1: Fill spray bottle with water, add Essential Oils, and shake well.

Mix 2: Fill spray bottle with water and Vinegar; shake well.

BRASS

1 part Water and 1 part Vinegar

Spray over brass and then polish with cloth for clean sparkling finish.

Mix: Mix water and Vinegar together in a spray bottle or put small amount into a bowl/ Wipe over the surface, shine, and polish with dry cloth.

CAR WINDOWS
Vinegar Spray, Water

Wet car windows with a hose. While the windows are still wet, spray with Vinegar. Wipe dry with newspaper if desired.

CARPET
Essential Oils 1 drop (as per blends), 1 tablespoon Bicarb

A carpet freshening powder is used the same way as commercial products, without giving you a dose of chemicals and at a fraction of the cost. Use Bicarb alone or combine it with a blend of Essential Oils to clean, neutralize, and deodorize.

Mix: Put 1 drop of Essential Oil for each tablespoon of powder into container. Shake well and sprinkle over carpet. Leave for 15-30 minutes and then vacuum.

Blends Suggestions
- Lavender for welcoming aromas.
- Lemon, Lavender (same of each) for clean citrus aroma.
- Eucalyptus, Tea Tree, Lemon (same of each) for antibacterial blend.

CARPET STAINS
50 ml Vinegar, ¼-cup Bicarb

To remove carpet stains, make a paste. Always test an out-of-sight part of carpet first.

Mix: Mix Bicarb with Vinegar and rub in the carpet stain. Leave on the stain until the paste is dry. (If possible leave over night). This can be followed by the carpet freshening powder.

CHROME
Vinegar spray

Spray over chrome and then polish with a cloth for clean sparkling finish.

COBWEBS
Spray Bottle, Lemon 10 drops, 500 ml Water

Clean away cobwebs. To inhibit cobwebs, spray the area with lemon spray.

COCKROACHES
1 part Bicarb, 1 part Sugar

A good cockroach killer is 1 part Bicarb and 1 part sugar. Spread it around the areas where you find cockroaches to get rid of them

COOKING SMELLS
Saucepan, Lemon 10 drops, ¼-cup Vinegar, Water or
Air Freshener Spray

Spray Air Freshener Spray around kitchen, if strong bad smells bring to the boil Essential oils, Vinegar and water on stove and boil for 5 minutes.

COMPUTER MOUSE
All-Purpose Cleanser

Spray All-Purpose Cleanser onto a cloth and wipe over the mouse. Be sure the cloth is not too damp and the electricity is turned off.

CUPS—COFFEE/TEA STAINED
All-Purpose Cleanser

Pour All-Purpose Cleanser into cup and rub with cloth. Rinse and wash as usual.

CUPBOARDS
All-Purpose Cleanser

Wipe out cupboards with All-Purpose Cleanser as suitable; always do patch test on surface in a remote area to ensure suitability.

CURTAINS
Air Freshener

Freshen up your curtains between laundering. The aromas will gently float through the area as the breeze moves the curtains.

Mix: Spray onto curtains.

CUTTING BOARDS
Vinegar Spray or All-Purpose Cleanser

Spray Vinegar Spray on the cutting board and leave for 1-2 minutes. Rinse and allow to dry. For removal of stains, cover with All-Purpose Cleanser, clean and rinse. Dry thoroughly.

DISINFECTANT

Ratio: 20 drops Essential Oil : 70 ml Vinegar : 180 ml Water

250 ml Spray Bottle
70 ml Vinegar
180 ml Boiled (Cooled) Water
10 drops Lavender Essential Oil
6 drops Lemon Essential Oil
4 drops Eucalyptus Essential Oil

Create an effective disinfectant to use around the house and spray onto most surfaces. Wipe dry or leave it moist behind toilets, fridges, washing machines, backs of cupboards, and along skirting boards—anywhere germs may harbor.

Mix: Mix in a glass bowl or jug; cool and pour into a spray bottle. Combine Vinegar with Bicarb (be sure to allow for the rising and foaming of Vinegar and Bicarb). Add water and Essential Oils. Shake well.

DISHWASHING LIQUID

Ratio: 10 drops Essential Oil : 250 ml Dishwashing Liquid

Dishwashing Liquid – Natural, Biodegradable
or make your own (see below recipe)
10 drops Essential Oil blend as below (Blend Suggestions)

Adding Essential Oils to your natural dishwashing liquid will give you a product that not only works as well as before but now has the additional benefits of the Essential Oils. Quick and simple, add this mixture to your bottle of dishwashing liquid or add 3 drops to your sink every time you wash up.

Mix: Add 12 drops of Essential Oil from the below blends to your biodegradable, natural dishwashing liquid (250 ml Bottle).

Make Your Own Natural Dishwashing Liquid

500 ml Sauce Bottle
5 tablespoons Soap Flakes or Soap (Grated) – Castle, Sunlight or Lux soaps
450 ml Boiled (Warm) Water
2 tablespoons Vinegar
2 teaspoons Glycerin
12 drops of Essential Oils from blends above

Mix together soap and water until soap is dissolved. Add glycerin, Vinegar, and essential oils. Shake well. This recipe will clean well, but will not foam, create bubbles or change water color. (You get used to it!)

DRAINS

1 cup Vinegar
1 cup Bicarb
10 drops Lemon Essential Oils

To reduce buildup in drains and eliminate unpleasant odors, use this recipe.

Mix: In a large bowl (to allow for rising and foaming of Vinegar and Bicarb), add Vinegar, Bicarb and Essential oils. Allow to foam and pour down drain. Leave for 5 minutes before flushing with hot water.

DRAWERS

Lemon 3 drops, Lavender 1 drop
Or All-Purpose Cleanser

To freshen clothing, drop Essential Oils onto a cotton ball and place in the drawer. Replace regularly for continued fragrance. Wipe out drawers with All-Purpose Cleanser to remove grime

DRYER

8 cm Square of Cloth,
4 drops Chamomile Essential Oils
4 drops Lavender Essential Oils

Mix: To fragrance clothes while drying, drop Essential Oil onto a small cloth no bigger than an 8 cm square and place in dryer with clothes.

EYE GLASSES
Surface Spray or Dishwashing Liquid

Clean glasses look better and provide you better vision. Use the Surface Spray or Dishwashing Liquid to clean glass and frames. Rinse well and then wipe gently dry with newspaper, which is environmentally friendly and lint free.

FLOOR CLEANER

Ratio: 10 drops Essential Oils : a Bucket of Hot Water

Mop
Bucket
Dishwashing Detergent or Soap Flakes (or soap grated)
10 drops of Essential Oils as below (Blend Suggestions)

Mop the floors with a clean damp mop using one of the following blends. No need to rinse. You can use the dishwashing liquid blend instead of creating a new mix.

Mix: Add 10 drops of Essential Oils into a bucket of warm water with detergent or soap. You can premix the blends into another 12 ml Glass Bottle or simple drop directly into the bucket from the original bottles.

Blend Suggestions:
- Welcoming. Lavender 10 drops
- Bacterial. Lavender 5 drops, Lemon 3 drops, Eucalyptus 2 drops
- Kitchen. Lavender 4 drops, Lemon 4 drops, Tea Tree 2 drops
- Bathroom. Lemon 5 drops, Eucalyptus 3 drops, Lavender 2 drops.

FRIDGES

250 ml Spray Bottle,
250 ml Vinegar
250 ml Water
10 drops Lemon Essential Oil
or All-Purpose Cleanser, Bicarb

Your fridge is a great place to collect odors from cooked and uncooked food, spills and drips. You need to clean and deodorize on a regular basis. A quick way to deodorize is to place an open container of Bicarb in you fridge or freezer as it will absorb smells. Stir occasionally and replace every two months.

To clean your walls and shelves and give your fridge and freezer a fresh clean aroma, wipe with All-Purpose Cleanser on damp cloth or create warm water clean bucket if a thorough clean is required.

Mix: Mix Essential Oils, Water, and Vinegar into Spray Bottle for regular use or in a bucket (with warm water if required).

FLY SCREENS
Air Freshener

Fly screens can become dirty very quickly and become a source of dust and allergies if not cleaned regularly.

Mix 1: If the screen can be removed, remove it and hose clean. Then spray with Air Freshener of choice. Allow screens to dry and return them.

Mix 2: If you would prefer not to remove or can't remove the screen, then vacuum it with a brush attachment and spray with Air Freshener of choice.

GLASS

Ratio: 10 Essential Oil : 250 ml Vinegar : 200 ml Water

500 ml Spray Bottle
250 ml Vinegar
250 ml Boiled (Warm) Water
10 drops Lemon Essential Oil

Glass shines up beautifully when cleaned and then wipe dry with newspaper, which is environmentally friendly and lint free.

Mix: In a spray bottle, blend water with 250 ml Vinegar and Lemon Essential Oil. Shake well.

Spray on mirrors and wipe with damp cloth or newspaper, then wipe dry with newspaper.

GLASSES – DRINKING

Ratio: *500 ml Vinegar : 1 liter Hot Water*

Use this when glasses get foggy and dull to create sparkling clean glasses.

Mix: In bowl (or sink), mix Vinegar and water. Soak glasses for 3-5 minutes. Rinse and wipe dry, or allow to drip dry.

GROUT

Vinegar

Clean grout by letting full-strength white distilled Vinegar sit on it for a few minutes. Then scrub with an old toothbrush.

INSECT REPELLENT

Ratio of Mix 1 and 2: 20 drops Essential Oil : 100 ml Water : 150 ml Base Oil

Mix 1
250 ml Spray Bottle
100 ml Water
150 ml Base Oil (or any oil, such as olive, sunflower, etc.)
8 drops Lavender Essential Oil
5 drops Tea Tree Essential Oil
2 drops Eucalyptus Essential Oil

Mix 2
Remove 3 drops Lavender
Add 5 drops Citronella Essential Oil (not part of Essential 5 Oils)
Follow recipe as above

A natural insect repellent is good for all the family. As many insect repellents contain DEET, a harsh chemical that can cause skin and body reactions, this is an ideal solution to alleviate the use of a very harsh chemical. This blend may be used as a house spray; spray it around windows, directly into the air and behind fridges—wherever creepy crawlies hide.

For oil burners, use a blend of Essential Oils without water or Base Oil. This is ideal to reduce mosquitoes and flies in rooms.

Mix: Mix the water and Base Oil together and add Essential Oils. Shake well. These products will need to be shaken before each use as no dispersant was added (chemical found in products to stop the products ingredients from separating, a quick shake does the same thing).

IRONING SPRAY

500 ml Water
10 drops Essential Oil as below (Blend Suggestions)
or Air Freshener Spray

Make a spray bottle of any of the below Essential Oils. Spray on clothes, then iron.

Mix: in 500 ml of water add 10 drops of Essential Oil

Blend Suggestions:
- Refreshing blend for everyday clothes.
  Lavender 8 drops and Eucalyptus 2 drops
- Storage. For storage and inhibiting moths
  Lavender 5 drops and Eucalyptus 5 drops

LABELS

Tea Tree (neat)

Labels are easy to remove with Tea Tree oil placed directly onto the label or sticker. Wipe off sticker and glue. Leave on for several minutes and wipe off. Repeat and leave on for a longer period if you have a stubborn sticker or label.

LAUNDRY

Essential oils

Add 3-5 drops of favorite Essential Oil into softener compartment on final rinse.

LIGHT BULBS

2 drops Geranium Essential Oil
2 drops Lemon Essential Oil
Cloth

Wipe over cold light bulbs with cloth soaked with Essential Oils. Enjoy the aromatic fragrance as the bulbs heat up.

MICROWAVES
All-Purpose Cleanser

For daily cleaning or spot clean, use All-Purpose Cleanser.

For stubborn stains, use 5 drops Lemon Essential Oil, ½-cup hot water, and ½-cup Vinegar

Your microwave may be part of your daily cooking and it gets splashes and spills. To clean and remove odors from a microwave, use All-Purpose Cleanser for daily cleaning and for spills. For stubborn stains and thorough cleaning, use the following recipe.

Mix: Place in microwave a bowl combining water, Vinegar, and Lemon Essential Oil. Bring to boil. Boil for two minutes. While the steam and moisture are still (damp food will be loosened and easy to remove), wipe over all the surfaces with damp cloth and All-Purpose Cleanser.

MILDEW

Bucket
500 ml Vinegar
2500 ml Water
10 drops Lemon Essential Oil
8 drops Tea Tree Essential Oil
4 drops Lavender Essential Oil

To get rid of mildew and staleness, wipe down with a cloth or sponge mop. For small areas, use undiluted Vinegar with Essential Oils in a spray bottle. Leave on for two minutes if required before wiping off wiping of with cloth. For large areas, mix Essential oils, Vinegar, and water into bucket and wipe area. No need to rinse.

MIRRORS

250 ml Spray Bottle
250 ml Vinegar
10 drops Lemon Essential Oil

Mirrors and windows shine up beautifully when cleaned and then wiped dry with newspaper (environmentally friendly and lint free).

Mix: In a spray bottle, blend water with 250 ml Vinegar and Essential Oil. Shake well.

Spray on mirrors and wipe with damp cloth or newspaper; then wipe dry with newspaper.

MOSQUITOES

Mix 1
250 ml Spray Bottle
100 ml Water
150 ml Base Oil (any oil: olive, sunflower, etc)
10 drops Lavender Essential Oil
10 drops Tea Tree Essential Oil
5 drops Geranium Essential Oil
5 drops Chamomile Essential Oil

Mix 2
Remove 5 drops Lavender
Add 5 drops Citronella Essential Oil (not part of Essential 5 oils)
Recipe as above

Use as air spray to reduce mosquitoes. This may be sprayed onto surfaces and materials, such as lounges and outdoor furniture. Patch test first.

For oil burners, use a blend of Essential Oils without water or Base Oil. This is ideal to reduce mosquitoes and flies in room.

Mix: Mix the water and Base Oil together and add Essential Oils. Shake well. This product will need to be shaken before each use as no dispersant was added. (A dispersant is a chemical to stop the ingredients from separating. A quick shake does the same thing.)

MOTHS

To inhibit moths, drop oils of Lavender, Citronella, Camphor or Rosemary onto cotton balls and place between clothes.

MOLD

Bucket
500 ml Vinegar
2500 ml Water
10 Drops Lemon Essential Oil
8 drops Tea Tree Essential Oil
4 drops Lavender Essential Oil

To get rid of mold, wipe the area with a cloth or sponge mop. For small areas, use undiluted Vinegar with Essential Oils in a spray bottle. Leave on for two minutes if required before wiping off with a cloth For large areas, mix Essential oils, Vinegar, and water into bucket; wipe area. No need to rinse!

OVEN CLEANER

Water
Bicarb Shaker
Vinegar Spray
Dishwashing Liquid

Spray or wipe oven surfaces with water. While surfaces are still damp, sprinkle Bicarb onto them. If surface is vertical, sprinkle Bicarb onto damp cloth and apply to surface. Allow to stay on surface for an hour (if very grimy, leave overnight). Spray with Vinegar and wipe over. Follow with warm water and detergent for final clean.

POLISHING

Bicarb Shaker

Stainless steel and chrome can be cleaned simply and effectively with Bicarb and a damp cloth. Sprinkle Bicarb over area and scrub in the direction of the grain. Always rinse and dry. If the surface is vertical, sprinkle Bicarb onto a damp cloth and apply to surface.

POTS AND PANS

¼-cup Bicarb, All-Purpose Cleanser

For burnt or crusted food, soak or boil water in pot.

Mix: Add Bicarb into the water and let stand until food loosens. (For a non-stick pot or pan, allow the water to boil but not to boil over.) Rinse and wash up. If scouring is needed (not non-stick), use All-Purpose Cleanser, or 1 part Salt to 1 part Bicarb before rinsing and washing up.

ROOM DEODORIZER

Air Freshener

Spray around room for clean fresh smell and to deodorize the atmosphere.

RUST

Lemon 15 drops, Vinegar

Remove rust by applying mix of one cup Vinegar to 15 drops Lemon and apply directly onto rust spot or soak large items in mix. Scrub with aluminum foil with shiny side up if required.

SHOES

Bicarb Shaker
2 drops Lemon Essential Oil
1drop Lavender Essential Oil

Freshen and renew the life of your shoes by reducing foot odor and staleness. Sprinkle the inside of shoes with Bicarb. (The Bicarb shaker is ideal.) Add Lemon and Lavender Essential Oils; tap out next morning

SHOWERS

Shower Doors and Curtains

Vinegar Spray

Spray with Vinegar onto dry doors or curtains. (Curtains may be washed with a cup of Vinegar as per manufacturer's instructions.) Allow to sit for one minute and rub over with sponge, releasing the hard water deposits. Rinse thoroughly.

Shower Head

½ cup Bicarb, 1 cup Vinegar

Into a plastic bag (sandwich bag size is brilliant), add Bicarb and Vinegar. Tie around the shower head and leave for one hour. Remove bag and turn on warm water. Wipe off showerhead.

SOAP

Essential Oils 10 drops: 500g Soap

Ratio: *Essential Oils 10 drops : 500g Soap*

Create a washer bag (made from sewing a washer into a small square bag with Velcro) and add oils to bath soap leftovers. This is a great idea for using up all the little bits of soap you end up with.

Blend Suggestions:
- Sleep Ease. Lavender 10 drops
- Cleanse and Go. Lavender 5 drops, Lemon 3 drops, Geranium 2 drops
- Beautiful. Geranium 6 drops, Lavender 4 drops
- Breath Ease. Tea Tree 4 drops, Chamomile 4 drops, Lavender 2 drops

SPIDERS

250 ml Spray Bottle
250 ml Water
20 drops Lemon Essential Oil

Clean away cobwebs. To inhibit cobwebs, spray the area with lemon spray.

STAINLESS STEEL CLEANER

Bicarb Shaker

Stainless steel and chrome can be cleaned simply and effectively with Bicarb and a damp cloth. Sprinkle Bicarb over the area and scrub in the direction of the grain. Always rinse and dry. If the surface is vertical, sprinkle the Bicarb onto damp cloth and apply to surface. If the item is badly stained, gently scour with table salt and then clean as above

STICKERS

Tea Tree (neat)

Stickers are easy to remove with Tea Tree oil (also Eucalyptus Oil) placed directly onto the sticker. Wipe off the sticker and glue. Leave on for several minutes and wipe off. Repeat and leave on for a longer period if you have a stubborn sticker or label.

Blend for Banishing the Burnt Toast

Finding a blend that will get rid of the burnt smell requires quick thinking. The smell may take a while to totally banish but in the meantime, why not harmonize the aromas?

In an oil burner, add 5 drops Lemon Essential oil and 5 drops Tea Tree, and place close to the toaster.

On the benches: In a bowl, add 5 drops Lemon Essential oil, 5 drops Tea Tree, and ½-cup warm water. Stir mixture and wipe off surface near toaster to release the aromas.

SURFACE SPRAY

Ratio: 15 drops Essential Oil : 60 ml Vinegar : 2 teaspoons Bicarb : 190 ml Water

250 ml Spray Bottle
2 teaspoons of Bicarb
60 ml Vinegar
190 ml Boiled (Warm) Water
15 drops of Essential Oils as below (Blend Suggestions)

This surface spray is great for quick wipe downs when an abrasive isn't needed. Use it on counter tops and any surface that needs cleaning using antibacterial cleaning agents without chemicals

Blend Suggestions:
- Germ Busting. Use wherever germs and bugs harbor.
  Lemon 9 drops, Eucalyptus 4 drops, Lavender 2 drops
- Aromatic. Welcoming and relaxing; ideal for bedrooms.
  Lavender 8 drops, Lemon 4 drops, Eucalyptus 3 drops

Mix: Add Bicarb, and then slowly add in Vinegar (to allow for rising and foaming of Vinegar and Bicarb). Mix together and fill with water. Shake well. Add Essential Oils from blends above and shake again. Always shake before use as no dispersant was added to keep the ingredients together (usually chemical-based additive). A quick shake will do the same thing.

TAPS

Bicarb Shaker or All-Purpose Cleanser

Stainless steel and chrome taps can be cleaned simply and effectively with the Bicarb Shaker and a damp cloth. Sprinkle Bicarb over the area and scrub in the direction of the grain. Always rinse and dry. If the taps are badly stained, gently scour with table salt and then clean as above. Use All-Purpose Cleanser on enamel and other surfaces.

TILES

Vinegar Spray, Bicarb Shaker, or All-Purpose Cleanser

To remove build-up on tiles and bathtubs, spray or wipe with Vinegar Spray and then sprinkle the area with the Bicarb Shaker, using a damp cloth. Rub as you would with a scouring. For a quick clean, use the All-Purpose Cleanser to wipe and rinse off.

TILE GROUT

1/3-cup Warm Water
1 cup Bicarb
5 drops Lemon Essential Oil

Mix: Mix Bicarb with warm water and Essential Oils to create a paste. Scrub into the grout with sponge or toothbrush. Rinse thoroughly.

TOILET

Vinegar

Deodorize the toilet bowl by allowing 3 cups white distilled Vinegar to sit in it for about a half hour before flushing. To make the toilet bowl sparkle, pour in a cup or more of Vinegar and let it sit several hours or overnight. Scrub well with the toilet brush and flush

Toilet Deodorizer

Drop a couple of drops of Essential Oil on the inside of the toilet paper roll. When it is turned, the aroma will be released into the air. Drop a couple of drops of Essential Oil into bowl (after cleaning) and do not flush.

VINEGAR SPRAY

250 ml Spray Bottle
250 ml Vinegar

A pure blend of Vinegar can be used by itself or as part of a cleaning system. This spray is ideal by itself for cleaning mirrors, glass and windows and with Bicarb for cleaning.

WASHING UP LIQUID

Ratio: 10 drops Essential Oil : 250 ml Dishwashing Liquid

Dishwashing Liquid – natural, biodegradable
or make your own (see below recipe)
6 drops Lavender Essential Oil
6 drops Lemon Essential Oil

Adding Essential Oils to your natural dishwashing liquid will give you a product that not only works as well as before but now has the additional benefits of the Essential Oils. Quick and simple, add this mixture to your bottle of dishwashing liquid or add 3 drops to your sink every time you wash up.

Mix: Add 12 drops of Essential Oil from the below blends to your biodegradable, natural dishwashing liquid (250 ml Bottle).

Washing Up Liquid – Natural; Make Your Own

500 ml Sauce Bottle
5 tablespoons Soap Flakes or Soap (Grated) – Castle, Sunlight or Lux soaps
450 ml Boiled (Warm) Water
2 tablespoons Vinegar
2 teaspoons Glycerin
12 drops of Essential Oils from blends above

Mix together soap and water until soap is dissolved. Add glycerin, Vinegar, and essential oils. Shake well. This recipe will clean well, but will not foam, create bubbles or change water color. (You get used to it!)

WINDOWS – FROST FREE

Vinegar Spray

Spray onto windows (ideal for cars) to help keep them frost free and clean

WINDOW SILLS

Air Freshener or Insect Repellent

Wipe over sills with Air Freshener of choice or use Insect Repellent if required.

WINDOWS

Ratio: 10 Essential Oil : 250 ml Vinegar

250 ml Spray Bottle
250 ml Vinegar
10 drops Lemon Essential Oil

Mirrors and windows will shine up beautifully when cleaned and then wiped dry with newspaper, which are environmentally friendly and lint free.

Mix: In a spray bottle, blend water with 250 ml Vinegar and Essential Oil. Shake well. Spray on windows and wipe with damp cloth or newspaper, then wipe dry with newspaper.

SECTION 6

First Aid and Common Ailments Solutions

THE BENEFITS OF NATURAL FIRST AID PRODUCTS

Creating a first aid kit and treating common ailments are great ways to realize the benefits of using Essential Oils.

Essential Oils bring their therapeutic benefits to the body as they are absorbed into the bloodstream via the skin or lungs. The aromatic fragrances can have a pleasing and powerful effect on our general well-being. As the Essential Oils enter the bloodstream, they take their healing powers to the part of the body that is in most need.

With First Aid and Common Ailments, you will make up more products that you use regularly, and this will bring even more benefits to you and your family.

I love creating my own first aid products. The process was quick and easy and I saved a lot of money, but the biggest benefit was that when I need something I could make it up quickly. If I needed a product for a one-off application, I could make up a small amount and I didn't have to buy a product that would then sit in the cupboard for years.

Originally I made up products only as I needed them but over time I found that there were products I used a lot or used over and over again, especially antiseptic cream (accidents and kids!). I now always have my Top 10 Kit products made up in a first aid kit along with band aids, bandages, and the like.

Using Essential Oils for first aid and common ailments is amazing; you really get to see the properties of the Essential Oils at their best.

The material in this book is not meant to take the place of diagnosis and treatment by a qualified practitioner. Seek medical advice as required.

THE COST COMPARISON OF YOUR FIRST AID STARTER KIT

When you first purchase high quality, 100-percent pure Essential Oils, you may think that you have spent a lot of money for such a small quality of oils, but a little goes a long way.

Essential Oils from a 12 ml bottle will provide you with 240 drops of Essential Oil. Compare the cost of buying the ten products.

Purchased Products (Generic or Cheapest Product Available)	Cost	Products Created Using Essential 5 Essential Oils and Household Products	Cost
Antiseptic Cream–30g	$3.75	Antiseptic Cream–100g	$3.00
Burn Gel–25 g	$5.95	Burn Gel–100g	$2.30
Chapped Lips–5g	$4.70	Chapped Lips–10g	.50
Headaches–24 tablets	$6.70	Headaches–10g	.75
Sunburn Gel–200 g	$5.70	Sunburn Gel–100g	$8.00
Insect Bites Cream–50 g	$7.50	Insect Bites–100g	$2.10
Cold Sores Cream–5 g	$8.10	Cold Sores Cream–10g	.80
Head Lice Treatment–250 g	$7.20	Head Lice Treatment–250g	$2.00
Eczema Cream–50g	$12.95	Eczema Gel–100g	$5.20
Sinusitis-24 tablets	$15.85	Sinusitis Blend	.80
TOTAL COST	**$78.40**	**TOTAL COST**	**$25.45**

RECIPES: FIRST AID AND COMMON AILMENT STARTER KIT

Ingredients List

You will need the following items to create one complete Starter Kit.

- ✓ Lavender Essential Oil
- ✓ Tea Tree Essential Oil
- ✓ Chamomile Essential Oil
- ✓ Geranium Essential Oil
- ✓ 4 50-ml Dark Glass Jars, New or Recycled
- ✓ 4 10-ml Dark Glass Jars, New or Recycled
- ✓ 2 200-ml Clean Bottles (Squirt or Pour), New or Recycled
- ✓ 43 ml Base Cream
- ✓ 354 ml Aloe Vera Gel
- ✓ 50 ml Base Oil

1. ANTISEPTIC CREAM

Ratio: 50 drops Essential Oil : 48 ml Base Cream

50 ml Dark Colored Glass Jar
48 ml Base Cream
20 drops (1 ml) Lavender Essential Oil
15 drops Geranium Essential Oil
15 drops Tea Tree Essential Oil

Use this antiseptic blend to assist in the healing of cuts and wounds. Use directly on the injury and cover with bandage or band-aid for quicker healing.

Mix: Into the glass jar, spoon in Base Cream until 2/3-full. Add in Essential Oils and mix with spoon. Fill jar with Base Cream and remix.

2. BURN GEL, MILD

Ratio: 50 drops Essential Oils, 48 ml Aloe Vera Gel

50 ml Glass Jar
48 ml Aloe Vera Gel
40 (2 ml) drops Lavender Essential Oil
10 drops Chamomile Essential Oil

When you have a burn, immediately apply cold water to area. Run water over the area for approximately 10 minutes.

For small areas, put a few drops of Lavender (neat) straight from the bottle onto area and follow with an ice pack. For large areas, apply blend above. I have this made up in fridge always because it works even better if the Aloe Vera Gel blend is cold. Apply clean gauze bandage and cover with ice pack.
ALWAYS SEEK MEDICAL ADVICE FOR A SEVERE BURN.

Mix: Into glass jar, spoon in Aloe Vera Gel until 2/3-full. Add in Essential Oils and mix with a spoon. Fill jar and remix.

3. CHAPPED LIPS

Ratio: 10 drops Essential Oil : 10 ml Aloe Vera Gel

10 ml Dark Colored Glass Jar or Container
10 ml Aloe Vera Gel
6 drops Geranium Essential Oil
4 drops Chamomile Essential Oil

Apply regularly to lips to keep them moist and smooth.

Mix: Into glass jar, spoon in Aloe Vera Gel until 2/3-full. Add in Essential Oils and mix with a spoon. Fill jar and remix.

4. COLD SORES

Ratio: 10 drops Essential Oil : 10 ml Aloe Vera Gel

10 ml Glass Jar
10 ml Aloe Vera Gel
4 drops Geranium Essential Oil
3 drops Tea Tree Essential Oils
2 drops Chamomile Essential Oils
1 drop Lavender Essential Oils

This blend can assist in reducing the severity of cold sores. Apply when the tingling, feeling starts. (If possible, apply to help prevent cold sores from forming.) Or apply directly onto the sore to keep it moist and reduce inflammation.

Mix: Into glass jar, spoon in Aloe Vera Gel until 2/3-full. Add in Essential Oils and mix with a spoon. Fill jar and remix.

5. ECZEMA GEL

Ratio: 50 drops Essential Oil : 48 ml Aloe Vera Gel

100 ml Glass Jar
48 ml Aloe Vera Gel
25 drops Chamomile Essential Oils
15 drops Lavender Essential Oils
10 drops Geranium Essential Oil

The Aloe Vera-based gel recipe has been formulated to alleviate the symptoms of eczema. It is gentle enough for inflamed skins (use half of Essential Oil drops for babies—and always spot test first). Apply gently onto inflamed or red areas.

Mix: Into glass jar, spoon in Aloe Vera Gel until 2/3-full. Add in Essential Oils and mix with a spoon. Fill jar and remix.

6. INSECT BITES

Insect bites are not dangerous, just very annoying. The itch, inflammation, and irritation become uncomfortable and stressful. Create a spray bottle using Mix 3 for larger slightly irritated areas. For poisonous insect bites, seek medical help immediately.

Mix 1
Ratio: Tea Tree
Tea Tree (Neat) – Directly on
Drop Essential Oil directly onto bite on a regular basis

Mix 2
Ratio: 25 drops Essential Oil : 48 ml Base Cream
50 ml Glass Bottle
48 ml Base Cream
12 drops Lavender Essential Oil
8 drops Tea Tree Essential Oil
6 drops Chamomile Essential Oil

Mix: Wash area to clean. Apply on area and repeat as necessary. Into the glass jar, spoon in Base Cream until 2/3-full. Add in Essential Oils and mix with spoon. Fill jar with Base Cream and remix.

Mix 3
Ratio: 26 drops Essential Oil : 150 ml Water : 50 ml Base Oil

200 ml Spray Bottle
50 ml Base Oil
150 ml Water
12 drops Lavender Essential Oil
8 drops Tea Tree Essential Oil
6 drops Chamomile Essential Oil

Mix: Wash area. Spray mix over inflamed area and repeat as necessary. Mix all ingredients and shake well before each use.

7. HEAD LICE HAIR TREATMENT

Ratio: 40 drops Essential Oil : 30 Base Oil : 170 ml Natural Conditioner

200 ml Bottle
170 ml Natural Conditioner
30 ml Base Oil
40 drops Essential Oil as below

Mix 1: *Geranium 10 drops, Lavender 4 drops, Eucalyptus 4 drops, Tea Tree 2 drops*

Mix 2: *Geranium 25 drops, Lavender 15 drops*

First, stun and remove head lice and nits from hair. Apply to hair and leave for 10 minutes. Do not remove. Place towel around the neck and divide the hair up into small sections. Comb through, wiping conditioner onto tissues after each comb. (This will contain lice and eggs and you don't want to return it to hair.) Continue until all hair is completed.

This will need to be done again before 7 days and then again 7 days later to break the breeding cycle since any eggs left may hatch and the process starts again

Mix: Pour conditioner into bottle. Add Base Oil and Essential Oils and shake well. (If you need this quickly and have no Natural Conditioner made up, use the cheapest bottle of conditioner from supermarket since it will be in hair for only about 20 minutes.)

8. HEADACHES

Ratio: 10 drops Essential Oil : 10 ml Base Oil

10 ml Glass Bottle
10 ml Base Oil
10 drops Essential Oils as below

Mix: Lavender 10 drops

To relieve headaches, inhale directly from the bottle, especially before leaving the bed in the morning. Massage onto pulse points, wrist, temples, and base of neck and across forehead. Drop 5-10 drops in bath or shower or use in an oil burner.

Mix: Pour Base Oil into a glass bottle, add Essential Oils, and shake well.

9. COLD AND FLU BLEND

Ratio: 10 drops Essential Oil : 10 ml Base Oil

10 ml Glass Bottle
10 ml Base Oil
6 drops Tea Tree Essential Oil
2 drops Chamomile Essential Oil
2 drops Lavender Essential Oil

Apply this blend to relieve the symptoms of colds and flu. Massage on face especially pulse points, behind and in front of ears, over cheek bones, and around the nose, forehead, and neck.

For inhalation, drop the oil into a large bowl of hot water (refer to Effective Applications for more details.)

Mix: Pour Base Oil into a glass bottle, add Essential Oils, and shake well.

10. SUNBURN

Ratio: 100 drops (5 ml) Essential Oil : 195 ml Aloe Vera Gel

200 ml Bottle (Squirt or Pour)
195 ml Aloe Vera Gel
50 drops (2.5 ml) Lavender Essential Oils
30 drops (1.5 ml) Chamomile Essential Oils
20 drops (1 ml) Geranium Essential Oil

Ouch, Sunburn! This blend is reputed to give relief to mild sunburns. Massage directly onto affected areas as often as possible.

Mix: Into glass jar, spoon in Aloe Vera Gel until 2/3-full. Add in Essential Oils and mix with a spoon. Fill jar and remix.

Love Using Candles?

Why not make Aromatherapy Candles?

Fat Candle
Essential Oil

First, light the candle and allow to burn for a few minutes, creating a pool of liquid wax around the wick. Blow out the candle and swirl the hot wax around until it is melted right to the edge (Burn out the whole candle, not just the small area in the middle.), and add your 5 drops of Essential Oils to this hot wax.

Use Lavender and Chamomile for relaxation; use Tea Tree and Geranium for stimulation.

RECIPES: A-Z OF FIRST AID AND COMMON AILMENT PRODUCTS

The following blends are given at the ratio of 1:1; that is 100 drops Essential Oil : 100 ml Base Oil, gel or cream, or 10 drops Essential Oil to 10 ml Base Oil, except when used for massage where the ratio will be 100 drops Essential Oil : 200 ml Base Oil.

I have made blends in 100 ml quantities for products that you usually need in larger quantities. For products you would use in a small quantity, I have made them up as 10 ml products. You can make them in any size bottle; just calculate the mix.

For example, if you purchase a 50 ml jar or bottle, halve all quantities; for a 30 ml jar or bottle, reduce your recipe to a third. If you use a 200 ml, jar or bottle, then double the recipe. In this way, you can make the size you like.

All blends are to be made into glass jars and bottles (except massage blends) because the strength of the Essential Oil in these products will be absorbed into any plastic bottles, compromising the effectiveness of the blend and breaking down the plastic bottle.

AFTER SUN GEL

Ratio: 100 drops (5 ml) Essential Oil : 195 ml Aloe Vera Gel

200 ml Bottle (Squirt or Pour)
195 ml Aloe Vera Gel
50 drops (2.5 ml) Lavender Essential Oils
30 drops (1.5 ml) Chamomile Essential Oils
20 drops (1 ml) Geranium Essential Oil

Ouch, Sunburn! This blend is reputed to give relief to mild sunburns. Massage directly onto affected areas as often as possible.

Mix: Into glass jar, spoon in Aloe Vera Gel until 2/3-full. Add in Essential Oils and mix with a spoon. Fill jar and remix.

ATHLETE'S FOOT

50 ml Bottle
48 ml Base Oil
30 drops Lavender Essential Oil
20 drops Tea Tree Essential Oils

With athlete's foot, the skin gets itchy and the areas between the toes become white, moist, and soft (spongy texture). This is a well known problem in gyms and pool areas.

Add 1 tablespoon to bowl or foot spa (wipe over when finished with disinfectant), and add warm water to cover feet. Soak for five minutes and pat dry, particularly between toes. After drying, apply Bicarb or cornstarch to dry feet.

Mix: Pour Base Oil into bottle, add Essential Oils, and shake well.

BLISTERS (FROM BURNS)
Lavender, neat

Do not pierce blisters! Where possible, allow the blister to stay intact. Put 1 drop of Lavender onto blister and hold on ice for at least 10 minutes. Pat dry gently, and then put on another drop of Lavender. Cover with gauze. Repeat 3-4 times on the first day. If blister is broken, treat as above, but when the burning sensation goes away, in 1-2 days, apply antiseptic cream and cover with gauze, bandage, or band aid.

BLISTERS
Lavender, neat

Do not pierce blisters! Where possible, allow the blister to stay intact. Put 1 drop of Lavender onto blister. Pat dry gently, and cover with gauze. If the blister is broken, apply antiseptic cream and cover with gauze, bandage, or band aid.

BOILS

10 ml Glass Jar
10 ml Base Oil
6 drops Lavender Essential Oil
4 drops Tea Tree Essential Oils

This blend can help draw out the infection in boils. Drop 4-5 drops of this blend onto gauze and apply over boil. Cover (overnight if possible). Repeat until the head of the boil appears and releases.

Mix: Pour Base Oil into a glass bottle, add Essential Oils, and shake well.

CIGARETTE BURNS

100 ml Glass Jar
95 ml Aloe Vera Gel
100 drops Essential Oil as below

Mix 1: *Lavender, neat*

Mix 2: *Lavender 80 drops (4 ml) and Chamomile 20 drops (1 ml)*

Immediately apply cold water to the area and run for approximately 10 minutes. For smaller areas, apply a few drops of Lavender onto the area followed by an ice pack. For larger areas, apply Mix 2. I have this made up in fridge always because it works even better if the Aloe Vera Gel blend is cold. Apply clean gauze bandage and cover with ice pack. ALWAYS SEEK MEDICAL ADVICE FOR A SEVERE BURN.

Mix: Into glass jar, spoon in Aloe Vera Gel until 2/3-full. Add in Essential Oils and mix with a spoon. Fill jar and remix.

CHICKEN POX

100 ml Dark Colored Glass Jar
95 ml Base Cream
40 drops (2 ml) Chamomile Essential Oil
30 drops (1.5 ml) Lavender Essential Oil
30 drops Tea Tree Essential Oil

To relieve the itchiness and inflammation of chicken pox, dab this blend directly onto inflammation.

Mix: Into glass jar, spoon in Aloe Vera Gel until 2/3-full. Add in Essential Oils and mix with a spoon. Fill jar and remix.

COLD AND FLU BLEND

Ratio: 10 drops Essential Oil : 10 ml Base Oil

10 ml Glass Bottle
10 ml Base Oil
6 drops Tea Tree Essential Oil
2 drops Chamomile Essential Oil
2 drops Lavender Essential Oil

Apply this blend to relieve the symptoms of colds and flu. Massage on face especially pulse points, behind and in front of ears, over cheek bones, and around the nose, forehead, and neck.

For inhalation, drop the oil into a large bowl of hot water (refer to Effective Applications for more details.)

Mix: Pour Base Oil into a glass bottle, add Essential Oils, and shake well.

CRADLE CAP

100 ml Glass Bottle
100 ml Base Oil
20 drops (1 ml) Lavender Essential Oil
20 drops (1 ml) Chamomile Essential Oil
10 drops Geranium Essential Oil

To assist in the prevention of and improvement of cradle cap, baby eczema, and dry skin and to use as an everyday moisturizer for your baby, massage directly onto skin or add 1 tablespoon into baby's bath. Be sure you have a firm hold on the baby because the oil will make the skin extra slippery.

Mix: Pour Base Oil into bottle, add Essential Oils, and shake well.

– First Aid and Common Ailments Solutions –

CUTS

10 ml Glass Bottle
10 ml Base Cream
10 drops Essential Oil blend (as below)

Mix 1: Geranium 4 drops, Lavender 3 drops, Tea Tree 3 drops, Base Cream

Mix 2: Geranium 4 drops, Lavender 3 drops, Tea Tree 3 drops, 500 ml Water

This antiseptic blend assists in healing of cuts and wounds. Use directly on the injury and cover with bandage or band-aid for quicker healing.

DERMATITIS AND ECZEMA FOR BABIES AND TODDLERS

100 ml Glass Bottle
100 ml Base Oil
30 drops (1.5 ml) Lavender Essential Oil
20 drops (1 ml) Chamomile Essential Oil
10 drops Geranium Essential Oil

To assist in the prevention of and improvement of cradle cap, baby eczema, and dry skin and to use as an everyday moisturizer for your baby, massage directly onto skin or add 1 tablespoon into baby's bath. Be sure you have a firm hold on the baby because the oil will make the skin extra slippery.

Mix: Pour Base Oil into bottle, add Essential Oils, and shake well.

ECZEMA GEL

100 ml Glass Jar
95 ml Aloe Vera Gel
40 drops (2 ml) Chamomile Essential Oils
28 drops Lavender Essential Oils
12 drops Geranium Essential Oil

The Aloe Vera-based gel recipe has been formulated to alleviate the symptoms of eczema. It is gentle enough for inflamed skins (use half of Essential Oil drops for babies—and always spot test first). Apply gently onto inflamed or red areas.

Mix: Into glass jar, spoon in Aloe Vera Gel until 2/3-full. Add in Essential Oils and mix with a spoon. Fill jar and remix.

HICCUPS

1 drop Chamomile Essential Oil

Drop Essential Oil into brown paper bag and inhale.

Synergy of Bases

If you love mixing products or want an even better product, mixing your bases can give you a synergy. As they combine, the different properties of the Base Oils give even more benefits and that's on top of the benefits of the Essential Oils.

GRAZES

100 ml Glass Jar
95 ml Base Cream
100 drops Essential Oils as below

Mix 1: Antiseptic Blend

Mix 2: Basil 30 drops, Lavender 30 drops, Eucalyptus 40 drops, Base Cream

Mix 3: Geranium 40 drops, Lavender 30 drops, Tea Tree 30 drops, into 500 ml Water

This antiseptic blend assists in healing of cuts and wounds. Use directly onto injury and cover with bandage or band-aid for quicker healing.

Mix 1 and 2: Into glass jar, spoon in Base Cream until 2/3-full. Add in Essential Oils and mix with spoon. Fill jar and remix.

Mix 3: Blend Essential Oils into a bowl of warm water and gently clean graze. Use antiseptic cream after cleaning. Apply directly to injury and cover for quicker healing.

HAY FEVER

Directly from bottle
3 drops Lavender
2 drops Tea Tree

Use this blend in an inhalation (refer to Effective Application for more details), or place a few drops on a tissue and inhale as required

HEAD LICE

Head lice and nits are unfortunately a part of school children's life. They attach themselves to the strains of hair and live off the scalp. There are two different issues when treating head lice. First, the lice themselves need to be killed and removed; second, the nits or eggs need to be removed. Head lice lay eggs at the bottom of the hair shaft and can be hard to get off. The best way to get them off is combing with a special head lice comb (the metal comb is a lot more effective than the plastic) and conditioner, Essential Oil and Base Oil mix. This is an effective solution because the oil helps the eggs slip off and the conditioner and Essential Oils stun the head lice which can be removed from hair with comb.

HEAD LICE SHAMPOO

200 ml Bottle
200 ml Liquid Soap Mix
20 drops Essential Oil as below

Mix 1: Geranium 10 drops, Lavender 4 drops, Eucalyptus 4 drops, Tea Tree 2 drops

Mix 2: Geranium 25 drops and Lavender 15 drops

Use this first to kill the head lice. It is ideal for large infestations as first step in process. Apply to hair as you would normal shampoo. Massage though, especially onto the scalp and base of hair. Rinse out and treat with Head Lice Treatment.

Mix: Pour Liquid Soap Mix into bottle, add Essential Oils, and shake well.

HEAD LICE HAIR TREATMENT

200 ml Bottle
170 ml Natural Conditioner
30 ml Base Oil
40 drops Essential Oil as below

Mix 1: Geranium 10 drops, Lavender 4 drops, Eucalyptus 4 drops, Tea Tree 2 drops

Mix 2: Geranium 25 drops, Lavender 15 drops

First, remove head lice and nits from hair. Apply to hair and leave for 10 minutes. Do not remove. Place towel around the neck and divide the hair up into small sections. Comb through, wiping conditioner onto tissues after each comb. (This will contain lice and eggs and you don't want to return it to hair.) Continue until all hair is completed.

This will need to be done again before 7 days and then again 7 days later to break the breeding cycle since any eggs left may hatch and the process starts again.

Mix: Pour conditioner into bottle. Add Base Oil and Essential Oils and shake well. (If you need this quickly and have no Natural Conditioner made up, use the cheapest bottle of conditioner from supermarket since it will be in the hair for about 20 minutes.)

HEAD LICE DAILY SPRAY

200 ml Bottle
40 ml Natural Conditioner
20 ml Base Oil
140 ml Boiled (Cooled) *Water*
10 drops Essential Oil as below

Mix 1: Chamomile 6 drops, Tea Tree 4 drops

Mix 2: Geranium 6 drops, Lavender 4 drops

Use this spray each day to help prevent head lice. Alternate Mix 1 and Mix 2 because the lice get used to a product. This help make the hair uninviting to them.

Mix: Pour conditioner, Base Oil and water into bottle. Shake well. Add Essential Oils and shake again

HIVES

½-cup Baking Soda
10 drops Chamomile Essential Oils

Immerse yourself in a bath to relieve the symptoms of hives. Then apply the Antiseptic Cream.

Mix: Add baking soda to bath and dissolve. Add Essential Oils and stir to disperse the Essential Oils molecules.

INSECT BITES

Insect bites are not dangerous, just very annoying. The itch, inflammation, and irritation become uncomfortable and stressful. Create a spray bottle using Mix 3 for larger slightly irritated areas. For poisonous insect bites, seek medical help immediately.

Mix 1
Ratio: Tea Tree
Tea Tree (Neat) – Directly on
Drop Essential Oil directly onto bite on a regular basis

Mix 2
Ratio: 25 drops Essential Oil : 48 ml Base Cream
50 ml Glass Bottle
48 ml Base Cream
12 drops Lavender Essential Oil
8 drops Tea Tree Essential Oil
6 drops Chamomile Essential Oil

Mix: Wash area to clean. Apply on area and repeat as necessary. Into the glass jar, spoon in Base Cream until 2/3-full. Add in Essential Oils and mix with spoon. Fill jar with Base Cream and remix.

Mix 3
Ratio: 26 drops Essential Oil : 150 ml Water : 50 ml Base Oil

200 ml Spray Bottle
50 ml Base Oil
150 ml Water
12 drops Lavender Essential Oil
8 drops Tea Tree Essential Oil
6 drops Chamomile Essential Oil

Mix: Wash area. Spray mix over inflamed area and repeat as necessary. Mix all ingredients and shake well before each use.

NAPPY RASH

100 ml Glass Jar
95 ml Base Cream
20 drops Lavender Essential Oil
20 drops Chamomile Essential Oil
10 drops Tea Tree Essential Oil

This blend helps to prevent and heal diaper rash and rashes. It is gentle enough for use every time you change the nappy. Apply gently to area

Mix: Into glass jar, spoon in Base Cream until 2/3-full. Add in Essential Oils and mix with a spoon. Fill jar and remix.

RASHES

100 ml Glass Jar
95 ml Base Cream
100 drops Essential Oils as below

Mix 1: Antiseptic Blend

Mix 2: Chamomile 50 drops, Lavender 30 drops, Tea Tree 20 drops

Use the Antiseptic Blend or Mix 2 to assist with the inflammation of rashes. Keep the area dry and clean so the rash can heal.

Mix 1 and 2: Into the glass jar, spoon in Base Cream until 2/3-full. Add in Essential Oils and mix with a spoon. Fill jar with Base Cream and remix.

SAND FLIES

Lavender 1 drop (neat)

Apply directly onto bite

SHAVING RASH

100 ml Glass Jar
95 ml Base Cream
50 drops (2.5 ml) Lavender Essential Oils
50 drops (2.5 ml) Chamomile Essential Oils

This blend encourages the reduction of inflammation from shaving

Mix: Into glass jar, spoon in Base Cream until 2/3-full. Add in Essential Oils and mix with a spoon. Fill jar and remix.

SUNBURN

100 ml Glass Jar
95 ml Aloe Vera Gel
24 drops Lavender Essential Oils
16 drops Chamomile Essential Oils
10 drops Geranium Essential Oil

Ouch, Sunburn! This blend is reputed to give relief to mild sunburns. Massage directly onto affected areas as often as possible.

Mix: Into glass jar, spoon in Aloe Vera Gel until 2/3-full. Add in Essential Oils and mix with a spoon. Fill jar and remix.

WOUNDS

100 ml Glass Jar
95 ml Base Cream
4 drops Geranium Essential Oil
3 drops Lavender Essential Oil
3 drops Tea Tree Essential Oil

Use the Antiseptic Blend or Mix 2 to help healing of cuts and wounds. Use directly on the injury and cover with bandage or band-aid for quicker healing.

Mix: Into glass jar, spoon in Base Cream until 2/3-full. Add in Essential Oils and mix with spoon. Fill jar and remix; or use Antiseptic Cream.

USING OTHER ESSENTIAL OILS

Many Essential Oils are available on the market today, and many have complex and useful properties.

You can use the properties of the Essential Oils and the Base Oils to create the healing benefits of aromatherapy.

A larger range of Essential Oils would be needed to create a variety of Common Ailment products. Where possible I have tried to always give a recipe with the most commonly used Essential Oils, but sometimes specific oil is needed for its individual properties.

RECIPES: A-Z COMMON AILMENTS PRODUCTS USING OTHER ESSENTIAL OILS

ARTHRITIS, RHEUMATOID

100 ml Glass Bottle
95 ml Base Oil
40 drops Lavender Essential Oil
30 drops Eucalyptus Essential Oil
30 drops Cedarwood Essential Oil

To help relieve the symptoms associated with rheumatoid arthritis, apply this blend to inflamed areas. If possible wrap gently in muslin to further relieve the swelling. Drop 1 tablespoon of this blend into bath and relax in warm water.

Mix: Pour Base Oil into a glass bottle, add Essential Oils, and shake well.

ARTHRITIS, OSTEOARTHRITIS

100 ml Glass Jar
95 ml Base Cream
40 drops (2 ml) Ginger Essential Oils
30 drops (1.5 ml) Black Pepper Essential Oils
20 drops (1 ml) Cedarwood Essential Oils
10 drops Cypress Essential Oils

Use this blend in conjunction with gentle exercise to help reduce stiffness associated with osteoarthritis.

Mix: Into glass jar, spoon in Base Cream until 2/3-full. Add in Essential Oils and mix with a spoon. Fill jar and remix.

BACK ACHE

100 ml Glass Bottle
95 ml Base Oil
50 drops (2.5 ml) Lavender Essential Oil
50 drops (2.5 ml) Rosemary Essential Oil

Massage firmly onto area to reduce aches and pains. If symptoms continue, seek medical attention.

Mix: Pour Base Oil into a glass bottle, add Essential Oils, and shake well.

CAR SICKNESS

Peppermint (Neat)

Put oil on handkerchief and inhale.

CUTS

10 ml Glass Bottle
10 ml Base Cream
10 drops Essential Oil blend (as below)

Mix 1: Geranium 4 drops, Lavender 3 drops, Tea Tree 3 drops, Base Cream

Mix 2: Basil 3 drops, Lavender 3 drops, Eucalyptus 4 drops, Base Cream

Mix 3: Geranium 4 drops, Lavender 3 drops, Tea Tree 3 drops, into 500 ml Water

This antiseptic blend assists in healing of cuts and wounds. Use directly on the injury and cover with bandage or band-aid for quicker healing.

Mix 1 and 2: Into glass jar, spoon in Base Cream until 2/3-full. Add in Essential Oils and mix with spoon. Fill jar and remix.

Mix 2: Blend Essential Oils into a bowl of warm water and gently clean cut. Use antiseptic cream after cleaning. Apply directly to injury and cover for quicker healing.

FOOT ODOR

10 ml Glass Bottle
10 ml Base Oil
7 drops Tea Tree Essential Oil
3 drops Sage Essential Oil

Take the time to soak your feet for relief from foot odors and give you back your bounce. Add four drops to a bowl of warm water and soak feet. Dust feet with Bicarb and 4 drops of this blend. Place 4 drops inside shoes overnight.

Mix: Pour Base Oil into a glass bottle, add Essential Oils, and shake well.

HANGOVER

10 ml Glass Bottle
10 ml Base Oil
4 drops Grapefruit Essential Oil
3 drops Sandalwood Essential Oil
2 drops Rosemary Essential Oil
1 drop Lavender Essential Oil

Oh dear! Had one too many? This blend may help reduce the symptoms of a hangover. Inhale directly from bottle. Massage onto temples and around neck. Add 5 drops to bath or shower on final rinse. Hangovers cause dehydration, so drink plenty of water before, during, and after the event to help ease the symptoms.

Mix: Pour Base Oil into a glass bottle, add Essential Oils, and shake well.

HAY FEVER

10 ml Glass Bottle
10 ml Base Oil
4 drops Chamomile Essential Oil
3 drops Lemon Essential Oil
2 drops Lavender Essential Oil
1 drop Orange Essential Oil

Apply this blend to help relieve the symptoms of hay fever. Massage on face especially the pulse points; behind and in front of ears; over cheek bones, nose and forehead; and around the neck.

Mix: Pour Base Oil into a glass bottle, add Essential Oils, and shake well.

HEADACHES

10 ml Glass Bottle
10 ml Base Oil
10 drops Essential Oils as below

Mix 1: Lavender 10 drops

Mix 2: Lavender 6 drops, Peppermint 4 drops

Assist in the relief of headaches. Inhale directly from the bottle, especially before leaving the bed in the morning. Massage onto pulse points, wrist, temples, and base of neck and across forehead.

Drop 5-10 drops in bath or shower; may be used in oil burner.

Pour Base Oil into a glass bottle, add Essential Oils, and shake well.

INFLUENZA

10 ml Glass Bottle
10 ml Base Oil
5 drops Tea Tree Essential Oil
3 drops Thyme Essential Oil
2 drops Lavender Essential Oil

This blend assists in relieving the symptoms of flu. For quick relief, inhale. (For children, do not cover with towel. See "Effective Methods" in Introduction Chapter for more details.) Rub onto chests, back and neck. Use in an oil burner, inhale, or add 1 tablespoon in bath.

Mix: Pour Base Oil into a glass bottle, add Essential Oils, and shake well.

INSECT REPELLENT

250 ml Spray Bottle
100 ml Water
8 drops Lavender Essential Oil
5 drops Tea Tree Essential Oil
2 drops Eucalyptus Essential Oil
150 ml Vegetable Oil (or any oil, such as olive, sunflower, etc.)

A natural insect repellent is good for all the family. As many insect repellents contain DEET, a harsh chemical that can cause skin and body reactions, this is an ideal solution to alleviate the use of a very harsh chemical. This blend may be used as a house spray; spray it around windows, directly into the air and behind fridges—wherever creepy crawlies hide.

Spray directly onto the body as a body repellent; if a thicker product is required for the body, omit the water.

Mix: Mix the water and Base Oil together and add Essential Oils. Shake well. This product will need to be shaken before each use as no dispersant was added. (A dispersant is a chemical to stop the ingredients from separating. A quick shake does the same thing.)

ITCHING

100 ml Glass Bottle
95 ml Base Oil
40 drops Lavender Essential Oil
40 drops Tea Tree Essential Oil
10 drops Geranium Essential Oil
5 drops Eucalyptus Essential Oil
5 drops Cedarwood Essential Oil

When the bugs bite and the skin gets inflamed, use the Antiseptic Cream or make up this blend for itching skin to relieve the symptoms. If needed, wash area first to remove cause of itching. Apply directly onto area.

Mix: Pour Base Oil into a glass bottle, add Essential Oils, and shake well or use Antiseptic Cream for relief.

MORNING SICKNESS

10 ml Glass Bottle
10 ml Base Oil
6 drops Peppermint Essential Oil
4 drops Ginger Essential Oil

Morning sickness! Afternoon sickness! Whenever!! Help relieve the symptoms associated with morning sickness. Inhale directly from the bottle, especially before leaving the bed in the morning. Massage onto pulse points, wrist, temples, and base of neck and across forehead. Drop 5-10 drops in bath or shower; may be used in oil burner.

Mix: Pour Base Oil into a glass bottle, add Essential Oils, and shake well.

NAUSEA

10 ml Glass Bottle
10 ml Base Oil
6 drops Peppermint Essential Oil
4 drops Ginger Essential Oil

Relieve the symptoms of nausea. Inhale directly from the bottle or massage onto pulse points, wrist, temples, and base of neck and across forehead. Drop 5-10 drops in bath or shower; may be used in oil burner.

Mix: Pour Base Oil into a glass bottle, add Essential Oils, and shake well.

PSORIASIS

100 ml Glass Jar
95 ml Base Cream
40 drops (2 ml) Bergamot Essential Oils
30 drops (1.5 ml) Lavender Essential Oils
30 drops (1.5 ml) Sandalwood Essential Oils

This blend encourages the reduction of inflammation from skin troubles such as psoriasis (not suitable for children under five years).

Mix: Into the glass jar, spoon in Base Cream until 2/3-full. Add in Essential Oils and mix with spoon. Fill jar with Base Cream and remix.

RASHES

100 ml Glass Jar
95 ml Base Cream
100 drops Essential Oils as below

Mix 1: Antiseptic Blend

Mix 2: Chamomile 50 drops, Lavender 30 drops, Eucalyptus 20 drops

Mix 3: Chamomile 50 drops, Grapefruit 40 drops, Rose 10 drops

Use the Antiseptic Blend or Mix 2 or Mix 3 to assist with the inflammation of rashes. Keep the area dry and clean so the rash can heal.

Mixes 1, 2 and 3: Into the glass jar, spoon in Base Cream until 2/3-full. Add in Essential Oils and mix with a spoon. Fill jar with Base Cream and remix.

SINUSITIS

10 ml Glass Bottle
10 ml Base Oil
4 drops Rosemary Essential Oil
3 drops Geranium Essential Oil
2 drops Peppermint Essential Oil
1 drop Eucalyptus Essential Oil

Apply this blend to relieve sinus symptoms. Massage on face especially pulse points, behind and in front of ears, over cheek bones, and around the nose, forehead, and neck.

For inhalation, drop the oil into a large bowl of hot water (refer to "Effective Applications" for more details.)

Mix: Pour Base Oil into a glass bottle, add Essential Oils, and shake well.

TRAVEL SICKNESS

10 ml Glass Bottle
10 ml Base Oil
6 drops Peppermint Essential Oil
4 drops Ginger Essential Oil

Help relieve the symptoms associated with travel sickness. Inhale directly from the bottle, especially before leaving the bed in the morning. Massage onto pulse points, wrist, temples, and base of neck and across forehead. Drop 5-10 drops in bath or shower; may be used in oil burner.

Mix: Pour Base Oil into a glass bottle, add Essential Oils, and shake well.

WARTS

10 ml Glass Bottle
10 ml Base Oil
6 drops Lemon Essential Oil
4 drops Thyme Essential Oil

Use this blend to remove warts and inhibit the growth of new ones. Drop this blend directly onto wart every day for two weeks.

Mix: Pour Base Oil into a glass bottle, add Essential Oils, and shake well.

SECTION 7

Relaxation and Stress Relief Remedies

RELAXATION

"Time to relax? You've got to be joking." I have heard this time and time again and I know hard it is to fit it in. When my kids were little and my twins were about 6-months old (I had 5 under 5-years-old), I stopped taking time to relax. I decided it was a luxury that I couldn't fit in. Just getting the daily jobs done and looking after the kids was a challenge (some days more than others). So I didn't allow time to relax and I felt justified in not fitting it in. By the time the twins were about 9-months, I was a mess—both physically and mentally—but I just kept plodding along, thinking this is life with kids.

Then I saw a friend I hadn't seen for several months. She commented on how frazzled I looked and said I had looked so much calmer last time she had seen me. What had changed? She then went on to say that she wasn't commenting about my outer appearance (not that it was good) but she was talking about my inner calm. It was gone and I looked as if I was stressed to the maximum. I thought about it and realized the workload and the outside stresses hadn't changed; only I had unconsciously decided I didn't need to spend time on me. I had decided that "relaxing" was just a luxury I couldn't afford so I had stopped. I had lost myself in the nappies, sleepless nights, kids, cooking, and cleaning, I decided I had to find time for myself again.

Now finding time was hard. When could I get some time that was peaceful and relaxing? I heard of people getting up early in the morning. Ha! Not me. I get up only when I have to (not a morning person), so I decided it had to be at night before I went to bed. So after the night feed, around 10 p.m., instead on dropping in bed, I would take 10 minutes to a half hour for me. I tried to do this every night, usually did the 10 minutes but averaged 3–4 times a week for a whole half an hour. I would have an aromatic bath, meditate, light some candles, or listen to some music. Then I would go to bed and sleep soundly until the next feed, usually between 3-5 a.m. It took about a week of doing this for me to really feel the benefits, and everyone in the house benefitted because I wasn't so stressed. I seemed to get more done and looked forward to this every night. I refused to allow any excuses for not taking the time, and sometimes I even used it as an incentive to get jobs done that I didn't like.

Now the kids are older. I know I can change the time around but I have found that nights (being a night owl) are the best time for my relaxation—even if I don't go directly to bed and stay up later (I don't have early morning feeds and can sleep in a little longer :-).

By making my own relaxation products, I could adjust them to what I wanted and vary them to suit my moods. For example, I would use different oils for relaxing, for sleep, and for stress or meditation. These I will show you in this section along with great ideas and applications.

STRESS CONTROL

Stress in the right doses gets you out of bed in the morning and keeps you going. Not enough makes you feel flat, but give yourself too much stress and you are doing major damage to your life, your body, your family, your relationships and your mental state.

The level of stress that people can cope with is different. I seem to have a high threshold of coping (in the environment I am in), but I might not cope in a different home situation or work environment. Someone else might find my lifestyle stressful. We all have times that we can't cope (some days more than other). You need to accept and acknowledge them and try to relieve them somehow. Is there something you can change? If not, what can you do to help yourself cope?

Relaxation techniques are one way to relieve stress but there are other ways as well. I have a list of some solutions using Essential Oils and some other ideas that cost you nothing. They don't damage the environment, your health, or others' happiness or cause them stress.

Remember, you need to work out how much you can deal with Don't compare yourself to others because you will always find someone who is or seems to be coping better. Accept your personal level. Before you push past your limit, try to relieve some of your stress, allowing yourself to cope when the next stress factor hits. Let's face it—there will always be another wave.

How you deal with stress defines your life; it is not a measure of how someone else would deal with it. Life wouldn't be worth living without the ups and downs.

THE BENEFIT OF RELAXATION AND STRESS RELIEF

The benefits of making your own products for relaxation and stress relief are simple and effective.

You need to stop, whether for a quick one minute to do a deep breathing exercise, inhale a distress blend, or enjoy a one-hour massage. The choices you make are entirely up to you depending on your life.

Not everyone can have a weekly massage but you must allow time for yourself. I love massages but many times when the kids were little the budget and responsibilities didn't allow for it. However, it was great to get one from my husband and to give one also. Now the kids are older and I get one from them occasionally. This may not be a professional massage but sometimes it is just as enjoyable and relaxing.

Taking the time to light some candles, put on an oil burner, or do some meditation or exercise might seem to take away your time from something else, but in the long run your time becomes more productive.

THE COST COMPARISON OF YOUR RELAXATION AND STRESS RELIEF KIT

When you first purchase high quality, 100-percent pure Essential Oils, you may think that you have spent a lot of money for such a small quality of oils, but a little goes a long way.

Essential Oils from a 12 ml bottle will provide you with 240 drops of Essential Oil. Compare the cost of buying the ten products.

Purchased Products (Generic or Cheapest Product Available)	Cost	Products Created Using Essential 5 Essential Oils and Household Products	Cost
Body Oil–100 ml	$29.95	Body Oil–100 ml	$6.00
100-percent Pure Essential Oil Blend (More expensive pre–blended)	$24.95	100-percent Pure Essential Oil Blend (Mixed your own blend)	$19.00
10-percent Pure Essential Oil Blend	$16.95	10 percent Pure Essential Oil Blend	$2.50
Face Spray– 15 ml	$12.50	Face Spray–15 ml	$1.25
Bath Salts –200gr	$9.95	Bath Salts–200gr	$3.00
TOTAL COST	**$94.30**	**TOTAL COST**	**$31.75**

– Relaxation and Stress Relief Remedies –

The Essential 5 products are multi usable and can be used for many applications. See "Effective Applications for You" on the following pages.

For example
- Atomizers
- Bathing
- Bath Salts
- Bath Bomb
- Bath
- Bed Time
- Direct Application
- Footbath
- Humidifiers
- Inhalation
- Massage
- Meditation
- Oil Burners and Diffusers
- Room Spray
- Shower

RELAXATION AND STRESS RELIEF ESSENTIAL 4 BLENDS

We have set this chapter up a bit different from the others because most of the relaxation and stress relief techniques (applications) when used with different Essential Oils will give you a different result

For example, a warm bath with the Relaxation Release blend will relax and calm you; it is ideal for bedtime. However, a hot bath with the Stress Buster blend will calm the nerves and invigorate you.

These blends are formulated in 10-drop blends.
Multiply to create blends.
For example, the Body Oil needs 100 drops so you multiply the blend by 10; the Bath Bombs need 20 drops, so you multiply by 2.

RELAXATION RELEASE AND WIND DOWNBLEND
5 drops Lavender, 3 drops Chamomile, 2 drops Geranium

RELAX AND UPLIFT BLEND
4 drops Geranium, 2 drops Chamomile, 2 drops Lavender, 2 drops Lemon

CALM DOWN STRESS BUSTER BLEND
7 drops Chamomile, 3 drops Lavender

UPLIFTING DE-STRESS DELIGHT BLEND
6 drops Chamomile, 2 drops Lavender 2 drops Lemon

EFFECTIVE APPLICATIONS FOR YOU

There are many different ways to use Essential Oils and blends for relaxation and stress relief.

Atomizers

Atomizers are for air fresheners or to spray onto your face to refresh (usually a smaller bottle around 10–15ml). Using an atomizer is a quick way to pick you up and give you a refreshing mist of aroma. Always use glass bottles and use 1:20 ratio of Essential Oil and spring or distilled water.

Bathing

If you want to make your bath more than a cleaning process, you can change the ambience of the bathroom and relax and unwind. Light some candles. Add relaxing oils to your bath: warm to relax and hot to revitalize. Add 6-10 drops of 100 percent Essential Oil blend, Bath Oil, Bath Salts, Bath Bombs or Bath Bag to a full bath. Agitate the water to disperse the oil evenly before entering the water.

Bath Salts

Relax with these delightful aromas and allow the properties of Epsom Salts and pure Essential Oils assist your body's recovery.

Bath Bombs

Combine the natural fizz of Bicarb that stimulates your mind and body with the wonderful properties of pure Essential Oils to create bath bombs. Bath bombs will help the body and mind and are fun for the whole family

Bath Oil

Add to your bath to moisturize your skin and release the aromatic fragrance to add luxury and suppleness.

Bed Time Ritual

On going to bed, make sure you leave time for yourself and leave your problems out of the bed. Have a bath. Put on an oil burner and allow the beautiful aromas to help you let go. Turn on some relaxing music to complete a tranquil atmosphere.

Blends

Whether 100-percent pure Essential Oil or a diluted 10-percent Essential Oil blend, blends are used in many applications. Remember your 100-percent Essential Oil blend is not for use on your body; it must be a diluted blend for body usage.

The 100-percent Essential Oil blends are ideal for oil burners, foot spas, baths, inhalations, and meditation.

The 10-percent Essential Oil blends are diluted for topical applications such as pulse points, compresses and candles. (See 10-percent Essential Oil blend recipe for information.)

Breathing 1-Minute Stress Buster

Only have a few minutes? Use this simple stress buster exercise and inhalation to calm the body and mind. Sit straight in a chair and tense up every muscle in your body. Squeeze your eyes shut and take in a big breath in. Hold for 2-4 seconds and release the breath and the muscles at the same time. Repeat 3-5 times, depending on the time you have available. As you breathe in, inhale the 100-percent Essential Oils for stress relief

Compress

Drop 10-percent Essential Oil blend into approximately 250 ml Water. Stir or agitate the water to thoroughly disperse the oil. Place a cloth or gauze into the water, squeeze out, and then place onto the affected area.

Use a cold compress for headaches, migraines, eye aches, and tension. Leave the compress in place for approximately 20 minutes or until the compress gets warm.

Candles

Rub your 10-percent Essential Oil blend onto a candle. Apply oil up the sides of the candle. Use your candle after applying as the Essential Oils will start to evaporate. If you are using a candle in a jar or using a fat candle, add the Essential Oil to the hot wax. Blow out the flame—Essential Oils are flammable— and drop in Essential Oil blend. Relight candle.

Direct Application

Although direct application of 100-percent Essential Oils is not recommended (with the exception of Lavender and Tea Tree), you can use 10-percent Essential Oil blends on the body.

Exercise

To some "exercise" is a dirty word; the thought of exercising fills them with dread. To others, it's a way of life. You must learn to do some sort of exercise very day. This doesn't have to be going to the gym or running if you're not into that, but you must make a conscious effort every day to do some exercise that makes your heart beat faster. You will be more relaxed and less stressed because your body will love the heart working hard.
This can be simply with you music on. Instead of just cleaning up, move around and dance with your vacuum. I know it's going to be a funny sight, but that's half the benefit. Go for a walk with your family, join a yoga or tai chi class, go swimming—it doesn't matter as long as you get going and move.

Footbath

A footbath is a wonderful way to relax and unwind. Either use a foot spa or create your own with a basin, marbles, warm water and relaxing Essential Oils.

When you use a foot spa, fill as per instructions and then add 4 drops of 100-percent Essential Oil.

When you use a basic, choose one large enough for your soles to lie flat on the bottom. Place large round stones or marbles on bottom of bowl. Fill 2/3 of the basin with warm to hot water and add 5 drops of 100-percent Essential Oil blend. Agitate the water and roll the soles of your feet over stones for a mini massage. Soak for a minimum of 15 minutes.

Humidifiers

Add Essential Oils to the water and follow the humidifier's instructions.

Inhalation

Add 5-10 drops of 100-percent Essential Oil blend to a large bowl of boiling water. Stir quickly with a metal spoon (wooden spoon will absorb the oils). Place a towel over your head and the bowl and inhale gently. Do not put your face too close to the water since the steam will be too hot.

This application is an invaluable aid for relief of colds, sinuses, and headaches. It is also ideal to hydrate and cleanse skin and improve stamina. For a quick inhalation, add 1-2 drops of Essential Oil neat—not diluted—to a handkerchief or tissue and inhale.

Journal or Diary

It's amazing how de-stressing it is to write down and let go of the negative in the day and to be grateful and appreciate the positive. In a journal or diary, write down the negative and accept it has happened. Work out what you can learn from it and then write what you can learn as a positive. Finish with giving thanks for all the great things that are happening in your life.

Massage

Massage is one of the oldest forms of treatment. Using your Body Oil as an aromatic massage will leave you feeling wonderful for several days. Getting a massage from a massage therapist—or a long or quick massage from a friend—is one of the quickest ways to relax and take time out.

Oil Burners and Diffusers

Made especially to use with Essential Oils, oil burners and diffusers warm the oil and release the molecules into the atmosphere. With a burner, fill the bowl on top with tepid water and light the candle at the base. Drop 6-10 drops of Essential Oils in to the water to disperse. As the water it warms, the molecules of the Essential Oils will be released into the atmosphere. Use the diffusers per the recommended instructions.

Room Spray

Make a spray for your room for an aromatic atmosphere or for an ailment, such as sleeplessness or colds. This can be refreshing or enjoyable. Add 10-20 drops to a 250 ml Bottle of water; spray into the air.

Shower

Wash as usual and place 2-5 drops of your favorite blend on your sprayer and rub over your body as you stand under the running water. Breathe deeply and inhale the aromatic steam.

Quick Relief

Dab 10-percent Essential Oil blends onto pulse points for instant relief

Meditation

A great and very positive way to calm your body and mind is through meditation. Start by shopping around for some meditation CDs that will walk you through simple meditation practices and explain what you need. This is an ideal way to learn how to relax your body and your mind. With experience you will be able to relax with simple body exercises or visualization as you need them.

Music

Music is a great way to relax, whether using relaxation music before going to bed or when taking a shower or bath. Put on your favorite music when cleaning the house. It's amazing how much quicker and better you work with music playing. Using music for relaxing and stress means allowing the music to make you feel good and inspire you to either relax or calm down. Dark music that makes you angry or really sad is best for another time—not for this.

RECIPES: 5 PRODUCT RELAXATION AND STRESS RELIEF STARTER KIT

You will need the following items to create one complete set:

- ✓ Lavender Essential Oil
- ✓ Geranium Essential Oil
- ✓ Tea Tree Essential Oil
- ✓ Chamomile Essential Oil
- ✓ Lemon Essential Oil
- ✓ 1 100-ml Dark Glass Bottles, New or Recycled
- ✓ 2 15-ml Dark Glass Bottles, New or Recycled
- ✓ 1 15-ml Glass Atomizer, New or Recycled
- ✓ 1 200-gram Jar, New or Recycled
- ✓ 350 ml Base Oil
- ✓ Epsom Salts
- ✓ 3 tablespoons Bicarb

RELAXATION AND STRESS RELIEF ESSENTIAL OIL BLENDS

Use your choice of blend and mix according to recipe directions.

These blends are formulated in 10-drop blends so you will need to multiply to create blends. For example, Body Oil needs 100 drops so you multiply the blend by 10; Bath Bombs need 20 drops, so you multiply by 2.

RELAXATION RELEASE AND WIND DOWN BLEND
5 drops Lavender, 3 drops Chamomile, 2 drops Geranium

RELAX AND UPLIFT BLEND
4 drops Geranium, 2 drops Chamomile, 2 drops Lavender, 2 drops Lemon

CALM DOWN STRESS BUSTER BLEND
7 drops Chamomile, 3 drops Lavender

UPLIFTING DE-STRESS DELIGHT BLEND
6 drops Chamomile, 2 drops lavender, 2 drops Lemon

1. 100-PERCENT PURE ESSENTIAL OIL BLEND

Ratio: 15 ml Essential Oil

15 ml Glass Bottle
15 ml Essential Oils (Your Blend)

Creating a blend of Essential Oils gives you a synergy of the oils. That means the combined benefit of the oils is higher than the individual oils. Remember your 100-percent Essential Oil blend is not for use on your body; it must be a diluted blend for body usage. However, 100-percent Essential Oil blends are ideal for oil burners, foot spas, baths, inhalations, humidifiers, diffusers and meditation.

Mix: Add the total drops of each Essential Oil into the bottle. Shake gently to blend.

2. 10-PERCENT ESSENTIAL OIL BLEND

Ratio: 30 drops (1.5 ml) Essential Oil : 13.5 ml Base Oil

15 ml Glass Bottle
30 drops (1.5 ml) Essential Oils (Your Blend)
13.5 ml Base Oil

While creating a blend of Essential Oils gives you a synergy of the oils, blending it down with Base Oil allows you the versatility to use for body applications. The 10-percent Essential Oil Blends are ideal for pulse point or quick relief, compresses, candles, direct application, showers, and inhalations.

3. BATH SALTS

Ratio: 20 drops Essential Oil : 200 gr Epsom salt: 1 tbsp Bicarb

200 grams Epsom Salts
20 drops Essential Oil (Your Blend)
1 tablespoon Bicarb
1 teaspoon Food Coloring, Herbs, or Flower Petals for Coloring

Combine the properties of these truly amazing natural products to create a simple and effective bath product. Add your Essential Oils depending on your mood and desires and lets your troubles float away.

Mix: To the Epsom Salts, stir in Bicarb and coloring product (if required) and mix well. Add Essential Oil blend and mix again.

4. BODY OIL

Ratio: 100 drops (5 ml) Essential Oil : 95 Base Oil

100 ml Glass Bottle
100 drops (5 ml) Essential Oils (Your Blend)
95 ml Base Oils

Use this if you prefer to use body oil instead of a moisturizer cream. The Body Oil will give the skin a supple appearance and is ideal for dry skin or skin in harsh climates where even the loveliest of skin has a tendency to dry up. Apply all over body, or apply directly after your bath when your skin is still damp. Gently pat dry.

5. FACE SPRAY

Ratio: 20 drops Essential Oil : 1 ml Base Oil : 13 ml Water

20 ml Glass Atomizer Bottle
20 drops Essential Oils (Your Blend)
1 ml Base Oil
13 ml Water

A refreshing face spray will give you an instant pick-me-up. It allows you to absorb the oils quickly at home or take your face spray in your purse and use it at times of daily stress.

Mix: Combine Essential Oils, Base Oil and water in atomizer and shake gently to combine all ingredients. This product will need to be shaken before each use as no dispersant was added. (A dispersant is a chemical to stop the ingredients from separating. A quick shake does the same thing.)

– Relaxation and Stress Relief Remedies –

RECIPES: A-Z OF RELAXATION AND STRESS RELIEF

If you are looking at this section and thinking there are not many products to use for Relaxation and Stress, remember that these products can be used in a multitude of way. At the end of each product are ways to use it to give you true benefits. For example, it's no use having bath oil if you don't have a bath but if you understand that you can also use it for massage and body moisturizing, you can also have different bottles with different Essential Oil blends. Use the one that suits your needs.

100-PERCENT PURE ESSENTIAL OIL BLEND

15 ml Glass Bottle
15 ml Essential Oils (Your Blend)

Creating a blend of Essential Oils gives you a synergy of the oils. That means the combined benefit of the oils is higher than the individual oils.

Remember your 100-percent Essential Oil blend is not for use on your body; it must be a diluted blend for body usage.

Mix: Add the total drops of each Essential Oil into the bottle. Shake gently to blend.

Uses
Oil burners, foot spas, baths, inhalations, humidifiers, diffusers and meditation.

10-PERCENT ESSENTIAL OIL BLEND

15 ml Glass Bottle
30 drops (1.5 ml) Essential Oils (Your Blend)
13.5 ml Base Oil

While creating a blend of Essential Oils gives you a synergy of the oils, blending it down with Base Oil allows you the versatility to use for body applications.

Uses
Pulse point or quick relief, compresses, candles, direct application, showers, and inhalations.

BATH BOMBS

160 grams Bicarb
40 gram of Citric Acid
20 drops Essential Oil (Your Blend)
1 tablespoon Base Oil
1 teaspoon Food Coloring, Herbs, Flower Petals for Coloring

Combining the natural fizz of Bicarb, that invigorates your mind and body with the wonderful properties of pure Essential Oils to create bath bombs that help the body and mind and are fun for the whole family.

Mix: Combine all dried ingredients in a bowl add Essential Oils 5 drops at a time and mix extremely well and then add Base Oil. If required add more Base Oil, your mixture should hold together into a basic shape. Press mixture into mold and allow to set for 2-3 hours. Press out and store in air tight container.

Uses
Baths, Foot Baths
100 ml (5ml) Essential Oils (Your Blend)
195 ml Base Oil

Enjoy the luxury of bathing with oil and the way it gives moisture to your skin and relaxes you. Use warm water to relax and hotter water to stimulate.

Mix: Pour Base Oil into bottle and add Essential Oil blend mix thoroughly and use.

USES
Bathing, Foot Bath, Massage, Moisturizing

BATH OIL - DISSOLVING

200 ml Bottle
100 ml (5ml) Essential Oils (Your Blend)
30 ml Base Oil
160 ml Vodka

Love oil and baths and the way it gives moisture to your skin and relaxes you but don't like the oil ring after? How about bath oil without the oil ring?

This blend will nearly dissolve completely in the bath water. A little goes a long way so don't go overboard. Add to your bath, and enjoy the aromas for relaxations and stress relief.

Mix: Mix together the Essential Oils and Vodka, stirring the mixture slowly to disperse all the Essential Oil droplets. Allow the mixture to stand for 2-3 days in a cool dark place. Then add water. Allow the mixture to stand for another 2-3 days in a cool dark place. Then you may use it. While you can make it in all one go, you'll make for a better product if you follow this time line.

BATH SALTS

200 grams Epsom Salts
20 drops Essential Oil (Your Blend)
1 tablespoon Bicarb
1 teaspoon Food coloring, herbs, or flower petals for coloring

Combine the properties of these truly amazing natural products to create a simple and effective bath product. Add your Essential Oils depending on your mood and desires and let your troubles float away.

Mix: To the Epsom Salts, stir in Bicarb and coloring product (if required). Mix well. Then add Essential Oil blend and mix again.

Uses
Bathing, Foot Bath, Prior to Massage for Muscle Relief

BODY OIL

100 ml Glass (or Plastic) Bottle
100 drops (5 ml) Essential Oils (Your Blend)
95 ml Base Oils

Use this if you prefer to use body oil instead of a moisturizer cream. The Body Oil will give the skin a supple appearance and is ideal for dry skin or skin in harsh climates where even the loveliest of skin has a tendency to dry up. Apply all over body, or apply directly after your bath when your skin is still damp. Gently pat dry.

Mix: Pour Base Oil into bottle and add Essential Oils. Mix well.

Uses
Moisturizing, Massage, Showering, Room Spray (Add 2 tablespoons to water and shake well.)

FACE SPRAY

20 ml Glass Atomizer Bottle
20 drops Essential Oils (Your Blend)
1 ml Base Oil
13 ml Water

A refreshing face spray will give you an instant pick-me-up. It allows you to absorb the oils quickly at home or take your face spray in your purse and use it at times of daily stress.

Mix: Combine Essential Oils, Base Oil and Water in atomizer and shake gently to combine all ingredients. This product will need to be shaken before each use as no dispersant was added. (A dispersant is a chemical to stop the ingredients from separating. A quick shake does the same thing.)

SECTION 8

Skin Care Sensations

THE BENEFITS OF CHEMICAL-FREE SKINCARE

As you can see, one of the benefits of making your own skin care products is definitely price, but where you will really see the benefits is in the condition of your skin.

When I started making my own products I noticed my skin loved the benefits of the Essential Oils and the high quality base products, and it looked so much better.

What I found was that I didn't react to anything in the blends because there were no chemicals to irritate my skin. If a blend seemed too strong on my skin, I just added more base product to reduce the strength of it; this made the blend lighter. I found this ideal for teenagers. When they first start using their own products, they usually have a tendency to be heavy handed and their skin is extra sensitive (hormonal). I found it was an ideal solution and over time if they felt the product wasn't doing its job (i.e. not a clean feeling), I then increased it to the original blend ratios.

When you put your first homemade mask on your face, you will be delighted at how it feels on your skin and how your skin feels afterwards. You will wonder why you haven't done this before since your skin will really love the pure chemical-free benefits you apply to it.

Your skin is the largest organ on your body, it is always "out there." It lives through all the weather and climatic stress you put on it and still it recovers. Many people don't appreciate the wonder of their skin and how beneficial maintaining a healthy complexion can be.

Today most of the products on the market are made with chemicals to give them shelf life and texture. Some have known carcinogenics in them (cancer-causing properties), but we use them. The beauty industry is a multimillion dollar in industry, with everyone vying to get our money.

Instead let's make products that are wonderful to use, great for our skin type, and less expensive than store-bought products. Imagine your own products—made especially for you—that are beautiful and effective; they actually help your skin repair the elasticity and tone.

I found that I could make a simple cleanser, toner, and moisturizer for daily use and a scrub, mask, and other products for less regular use. They were quick to make and quick to use, saving me time and money. Perfect!

When using skin care products, there are products for general skin use, but it is beneficial to get a cleanser and moisturizer suited to your skin type.

The skin is usually categorized so you must choose the correct skin products to be used. Skin can be termed Normal, Oily, Dry, Combination, Acne, and Aged or a combination of several types. You can tell your skin type by looking at it in good light and noticing several different aspects.

OILY SKIN

Oily skin usually looks shiny and usually feels smoother. This type of skin is prone to more acne and blackheads. Oily skin has larger pores and oiliness may reappear after only a couple of hours.

DRY SKIN

Dry skin usually looks dull and is sometimes flaky and rough to touch. Without regular moisturizing, this skin feels tight, drawn, and prone to fine lines and aging.

NORMAL SKIN

Normal skin usually has a flat appearance, with a healthy glow. It is supple, smooth, and usually blemish-free.

COMBINATION SKIN

The most common skin type is combination skin, which usually has drier cheeks and oily chin and forehead (your T-zone).

ACNE

Acne skin needs to be treated with an antibacterial cream for the acne and a moisturizer for evening out the skin and helping to reduce the blemishes. Always seek medical assistance with severe acne since it's often the result of an internal imbalance. This imbalance needs to be corrected to help with the external healing of the skin.

SENSITIVE SKIN

Sensitive skin can be any of the different skin types. When making products for sensitive skin, halve the Essential Oils used in the recipe.

Replace the Essential Oils for Different Skin Types:

NORMAL	OILY	DRY	COMBIN.	ACNE
• Lavender	• Lavender	• Lavender	• Lavender	• Lavender
• Geranium	• Tea Tree	• Lemon	• Lemon	• Geranium
• Lemon	• Chamomile	• Geranium	• Chamomile	• Tea Tree
• Chamomile	• Geranium	• Chamomile	• Tea Tree	• Lemon

THE COST COMPARISON OF YOUR SKIN CARE STARTER KIT

When you first purchase high quality, 100-percent pure Essential Oils, you may think that you have spent a lot of money for such a small quality of oils, but a little goes a long way.

Essential Oils from a 12 ml bottle will provide you with 240 drops of Essential Oil. Compare the cost of buying the five Skin Care Starter Kit products.

Purchased Products (Generic or Cheapest Product Available)	Cost	Products Created Using Essential 5 Essential Oils and Household Products	Cost
Cleanser–125ml	$9.95	Cleanser–125ml	$2.00
Toner–125 ml	$9.50	Toner–125 ml	$1.50
Moisturizer–75ml	$12.95	Moisturizer–75ml	$3.20
Mask–100 g	$11.95	Mask–100 g	$2.45
Night Cream–200 ml	$10.95	Night Cream–200 ml	$1.95
TOTAL COST	**$55.30**	**TOTAL COST**	**$11.10**

RECIPES: SKIN CARE STARTER KIT

You will need the following items to create one complete set:

- ✓ Lavender Essential Oil
- ✓ Geranium Essential Oil
- ✓ Lemon Essential Oil
- ✓ Chamomile Essential Oil
- ✓ Tea Tree Essential Oil
- ✓ 2 100-ml dark glass bottles, new or recycled
- ✓ 3 100-ml dark glass jars, New or Recycled
- ✓ 5 ml Base Oil
- ✓ 185 ml Base Cream
- ✓ 5 ml Vinegar
- ✓ 95 ml Liquid Soap Mix
- ✓ 100 ml Aloe Vera Gel

1. CLEANSER

Ratio: 100 drops (5 ml) Essential Oil : 95 Liquid Soap Mix

100 ml Glass Bottle
100 drops (5 ml) Essential Oil
95 ml Liquid Soap Mix

Blend Suggestionss

Normal, Oily, Acne Skin Types
60 drops (3 ml) Lavender, 40 drops (2 ml) Lemon Essential Oils

Dry and Combination Skin Types
60 drops (3 ml) Lavender, 40 drops (2 ml) Geranium Essential Oils

Massage onto face, neck and décolleté and wash off with warm water and cloth (or cotton wipes). You will need to wipe 2-3 times, to remove all oil and grime from skin. Rinse again, tone, pat dry and moisturize.

Mix: Pour in Liquid Soap Mix into bottle, add to this your Essential Oils and shake well. For babies and children up to 2 years, half the quantity of essential oils.

2. TONER

Ratio: 40 drops Essential Oil: 5 ml Vinegar: 93 ml Water

100 ml Glass Bottle
40 drops (2 ml) Lavender Essential Oil
5 ml Vinegar
93 ml Water

Apply to cotton ball and gently wipe of face

Mix: Add Water and Vinegar to bottle and then add Essential Oil. Mix thoroughly. Shake well before each use as no dispersant is used. (A dispersant is usually found in commercial products to keep products from separating.)

Did You Know?

Natural skin care can be traced back to the 4th millennium BC in Middle East and China. The Egyptians are believed to have developed treatments for skin conditions.

Lead was used in skincare for hundreds of years, with the Ancient Greeks covering their faces in mixtures containing lead to whiten and cover blemishes. It wasn't until the late 1860 that lead was removed from skincare.

3. MOISTURIZER

Ratio: 100 drops (5 ml) Essential Oils: 95 ml Base Cream

100 ml Glass Jar
100 drops (5 ml) Essential Oil blend (as below)
95 ml Base Cream

Blend Suggestions

dr = drop

Normal Skin
30 dr Lavender, 30 dr Geranium, 20 dr Lemon, 20 dr Chamomile

Oily Skin
40 dr Geranium, 25 dr Lavender, 25 dr Tea Tree, 10 dr Chamomile

Dry Skin
35 dr Lemon, 35 dr Lavender, 20 dr Geranium, 15 dr Chamomile

Combination Skin
30 dr Lavender, 30 dr Lemon, 20 dr Chamomile, 20 dr Tea Tree

Acne Skin
35 dr Tea Tree, 25 dr Lavender, 20 dr Geranium, 20 dr Lemon

After cleansing and toning you will need to add moisture back to your skin (even oily) Use this blend daily before apply makeup or as part of the morning / evening skincare ritual.

Mix: Into glass jar spoon in Base Cream fill 2/3 of jar add in essential oils, mix with spoon, fill jar and remix

4. FACE MASK

Ratio: 10 drops Lavender: 100 ml Aloe Vera Gel

100 ml Glass Jar
10 drops Lavender Essential Oil
100 ml Aloe Vera Gel

Using the natural healing and restoring properties of Aloe Vera Gel, this mask draws impurities from the skin gently and without stressing the skins natural balance. Apply mixture evenly over face and neck. Leave on for at least 5 minutes (may feel dry and tight) and rinse with warm water, gently pat dry at apply a moisturizer cream or oil (suitable for your skin type)

Mix: Into glass jar spoon in Aloe Vera Gel fill 2/3 of jar add in essential oils, mix with spoon, fill jar and remix (note: the Aloe Vera Gel will go cloudy because of the Essential Oils)

5. NIGHT CREAM

Ratio: 50 drops Essential Oil: 2.5 ml Base Oil: 95 ml Base Cream

100 ml Glass Jar
30 drops Geranium Essential oil
20 drops Lavender
2.5 ml Base Oil
95ml Base Cream

Use this blend at night before retiring to deep moisturize your skin, allowing the oils to penetrate and rejuvenate the skin throughout the night, waking up to soft and supple skin.

Mix: Into glass jar pour in Base Oil and spoon in Base cream fill 2/3 of jar add in essential oils, mix with spoon, fill jar and remix

RECIPES: A-Z OF SKINCARE

BODY OIL

Ratio: 100 drops (5 ml) Essential Oil : 95 Base Oil

100 ml Glass Bottle
100 drops Lavender (5 ml) Essential Oil
95 ml Base Oils

This recipe gives you a great oil; use this if you prefer to use a body oil, instead of a moisturizer cream. Body is great to give skin supple appearance and ideal for dry skin or skin in harsh climates where even the loveliest of skin has a tendency to dry up. Apply all over body, for added directly after bath with skin is still damp and gently pat dry.

Mix: Add Base Oils to your Essential Oil. Blend and mix well.

CLEANSER

Ratio: 100 drops (5 ml) Essential Oil : 95 Liquid Soap Mix

100 ml Glass Bottle
100 drops (5 ml) Essential Oil
95 ml Liquid Soap Mix

Blend Suggestions

Normal, Oily, Acne Skin Types
60 drops (3 ml) Lavender, 40 drops (2 ml) Lemon Essential Oils

Dry and Combination Skin Types
60 drops (3 ml) Lavender, 40 drops (2 ml) Geranium Essential Oils

Massage onto face, neck and décolleté and wash off with warm water and cloth (or cotton wipes). You will need to wipe 2-3 times, to remove all oil and grime from skin. Rinse again, tone, pat dry and moisturize.

Mix: Pour in Liquid Soap Mix into bottle, add to this your Essential Oils and shake well. For babies and children up to 2 years, half the quantity of essential oils.

CLEANSING OIL

Ratio: 100 drops (5 ml) Essential Oil : 95 Base Oil

100 ml Glass Bottle
100 drops (5 ml) Essential Oil
95 ml Base Oil

Blend Suggestions

Normal, Oily, Acne Skin Types

60 drops (3 ml) Lavender, 40 drops (2 ml) Lemon Essential Oils

Dry and Combination Skin Types

60 drops (3 ml) Lavender, 40 drops (2 ml) Geranium Essential Oils

If you like the feel of oil and love the natural way it cleans as grime the use this oil base cleanser. Massage onto face, neck and décolleté and wash off with warm water and cloth (or cotton wipes). You will need to wipe 2-3 times, to remove all oil and grime from skin. Rinse again, tone, pat dry and moisturize.

Mix: Pour in Base Oil into bottle, add to this your Essential Oils and shake well.

FACE MASK

Ratio: 10 drops Lavender: 100 ml Aloe Vera Gel

100 ml Glass Jar
10 drops Lavender Essential Oil
100 ml Aloe Vera Gel

Using the natural healing and restoring properties of Aloe Vera Gel, this mask draws impurities from the skin gently and without stressing the skins natural balance. Apply mixture evenly over face and neck. Leave on for at least 5 minutes (may feel dry and tight) and rinse with warm water, gently pat dry at apply a moisturizer cream or oil (suitable for your skin type)

Mix: Into glass jar spoon in Aloe Vera Gel fill 2/3 of jar add in essential oils, mix with spoon, fill jar and remix (note: the Aloe Vera Gel will go cloudy because of the Essential Oils)

FACE SPRAY

Ratio: 20 drops Essential Oil : 1 ml Base Oil: 13 ml Water

20 ml glass Atomizer Bottle
10 drops Lavender Essential Oil
5 drops Lemon Essential Oil
5 drops Geranium Essential Oil
1 ml Base Oil
13 ml Water

A refreshing face spray gives you an instant pick-me-up; it enables you to absorb the oils quickly at home. Or take your face spray in your purse and use it at times of daily stress.

Mix: Combine Essential Oils, Base Oil and Water in atomizer and shake gently to combine all ingredients. Shake before each use as no dispersant (usually chemical based) was used in this blend to keep the oils and water from separating.

MOISTURIZER

Ratio: 100 drops (5 ml) Essential Oils: 95 ml Base Cream

100 ml Glass Jar
100 drops (5 ml) Essential Oil blend (as below)
95 ml Base Cream

Blend Suggestionss

dr = drop

Normal Skin
30 dr Lavender, 30 dr Geranium, 20 dr Lemon, 20 dr Chamomile

Oily Skin
40 dr Geranium, 25 dr Lavender, 25 dr Tea Tree, 10 dr Chamomile

Dry Skin
35 dr Lemon, 35 dr Lavender, 20 dr Geranium, 15 dr Chamomile

Combination Skin
30 dr Lavender, 30 dr Lemon, 20 dr Chamomile, 20 dr Tea Tree

Acne Skin
35 dr Tea Tree, 25 dr Lavender, 20 dr Geranium, 20 dr Lemon

After cleansing and toning you will need to add moisture back to your skin (even oily) Use this blend daily before apply makeup or as part of the morning / evening skincare ritual.

Mix: Into glass jar spoon in Base Cream fill 2/3 of jar add in essential oils, mix with spoon, fill jar and remix

NIGHT CREAM

Ratio: 50 drops Essential Oil: 2.5 ml Base Oil: 95 ml Base Cream

100 ml Glass Jar
30 drops Geranium Essential oil
20 drops Lavender
2.5 ml Base Oil
95ml Base Cream

Use this blend at night before retiring to deep moisturize your skin, allowing the oils to penetrate and rejuvenate the skin throughout the night, waking up to soft and supple skin.

Mix: Into glass jar pour in Base Oil and spoon in Base cream fill 2/3 of jar add in essential oils, mix with spoon, fill jar and remix

TONER

Ratio: 40 drops Essential Oil: 5 ml Vinegar: 93 ml Water

100 ml Glass Bottle
40 drops (2 ml) Lavender Essential Oil
5 ml Vinegar
93 ml Water

Apply to cotton ball and gently wipe off face

Mix: Add Water and Vinegar to bottle and then add Essential Oil. Mix thoroughly. Shake well before each use as no dispersant is used. (A dispersant is an ingredient found in commercial products to keep them from separating.)

SECTION 9

Hair Care Help

Your "crowning glory" is an important part of your appearance and your confidence. If your hair is oily, messy, or lifeless, it doesn't matter how well you dress: your appearance lacks the finesse of the "together" look. Why do you think there is the term "bad hair day"? If you're like me, that could be every day as I have curly hair that has a tendency to look messy.

I found I could change this with the right products and lots of expense, but I decided to find natural alternatives that didn't break the bank and could help my hair without filling it full of chemicals. I loved that I could cut down the expense of looking after my hair and have had hairdressers comment on the condition it is in. This allowed me to spend some of the savings on a good hair cut.

Essential Oils do not change your natural hair color but they can enhance it and bring out the shine. Essential Oils are fabulous for reducing oil, adding moisture, relieving dry scalps and psoriasis, treating head lice (see recipe in First Aid Chapter), and generally making your hair look and feel great. So add to that a great hair cut and, *voilà*, you can have a "Good Hair Day" every day.

THE BENEFITS OF LOOKING AFTER YOUR CROWNING GLORY NATURALLY

As you can see, cost is a major factor when using treatments and specialty products. I didn't save a great deal on shampoos and conditioners when I was buying the cheaper ones because I'm sure the kids were pouring half a bottle per shampoo on their heads. That was how fast we seemed to be going through it. What I found was that I was getting a good quality shampoo and conditioner for the same price as the cheaper shampoo I was buying. I also found that with the natural shampoos, I didn't need as many other products to keep our hair looking shiny and healthy.

I alternated between Natural Shampoo to Eggy Shampoo, making them in two-bottle batches. I found my hair thrived and so did my family and friends who used it. I know sometimes you just don't have the time or desire to make from shampoos or conditioners from scratch. That's fine. If you like, use a gentle natural baby product for your base and you will still receive the benefits of Essential Oils.

Where I really found the cost saving was when I used my after care products (for our house four females with long hair—you do the math). They worked well and they were very cheap.

A friend of mine found that the anti-dandruff treatment was effective and after a period of time she didn't need to use it any more. She then went on to the Natural Shampoo and Conditioner. This saved her money and alleviated the problem. Sometimes she finds it starting to return so she makes up a new bottle of anti-dandruff product and uses it until the problem is gone. By using natural products with no chemicals, your hair will thank you, and so will your hip pocket.

Hair can be categorized into Normal (balanced), Dry, Oily, Damaged or Dandruff, choosing the correct product can enhance and help repair your hair.

Hair in made on keratin the same as your nails and the outer layer or the skin and reacts to daily stresses, environmental exposure (sun, wind etc) and chemicals and the processes we use on it. The use of strengtheners, hair dryers, and harsh products can all be a factor in the hairs conditions. You can tell your hair type by looking at it and noticing several factors.

OILY HAIR

Oily hair usually looks greasy after washing and seems to attract more dirt. Washing only every 3-4 days is ideal.

DRY HAIR

Dry skin usually looks dull and usually frizzy and unmanageable. It is prone to look messy again shortly after styling. Weekly oil based treatments are ideal for this hair type.

NORMAL HAIR

Normal skin is easy to manage and looks shinny and bouncy with the minimum fuss. Can be washed daily if required but to ensure continued balance always clean well and maintain.

DAMAGED HAIR

Hair that lacks elasticity and is hard to maintain, while not dry or oily, is usually damaged hair. The hair type is more common than you realize with the amount of drying and chemical bases products added to own hair. This is usually only a temporary state that with the use of good products and less harsh handling can be reduced.

DANDRUFF

While this is not a hair type it is a cause of concern and needs to be treated. Treating your dandruff required patience and use of products especially designed to relieve the scalp of flakiness.

Replace the Essential Oils for Different Hair Types:

The skin is usually categorized allowing for correct skin products to be used. Skin can be Normal, Oily, Dry, Combination, Acne and Aged or a combination of several types. You can tell your skin type by having a look at it in good light and noticing several different aspects.

NORMAL	OILY	DRY	DAMAGED	DANDRUFF
Lavender	Lavender	Lavender	Lavender	Lavender
Chamomile	Chamomile	Geranium	Chamomile	Chamomile
Lemon	Geranium	Chamomile	Geranium	Lemon
Geranium	Tea Tree	Lemon	Tea Tree	Tea Tree

THE COST COMPARISON OF YOUR HAIR CARE STARTER KIT

When you first purchase high quality, 100-percent pure Essential Oils, you may think that you have spent a lot of money for such a small quality of oils, but a little goes a long way.

Essential Oils from a 12 ml bottle will provide you with 240 drops of Essential Oil. Compare the cost of buying the five Kit products.

Purchased Products (Generic or Cheapest Product Available)	Cost	Products Created Using Essential 5 Essential Oils and Household Products	Cost
Shampoo–250 ml	$1.85	Shampoo–250 ml	$1.00
Conditioner–250 ml	$1.85	Conditioner–250 ml	.50
Shine Treatment– 250 ml	$3.90	Shine Treatment– 250 ml	$3.00
Leave in Conditioner– 250 ml	$6.50	Leave in Conditioner– 250 ml	.45
Hot Oil Treatment– 15 ml x 3	$9.95	Hot Oil Treatment– 15 ml x 3	$5.00
TOTAL COST	**$23.95**	**TOTAL COST**	**$9.95**

– Hair Care Help –

RECIPES: 5-PRODUCT HAIR CARE STARTER KIT

Ingredients List

Your will need the following items:

- ✓ Lavender Essential Oil
- ✓ Geranium Essential Oil
- ✓ Lemon Essential Oil
- ✓ Chamomile Essential Oil
- ✓ Tea Tree Essential Oil
- ✓ 200 ml of Liquid Soap Mix
- ✓ 142 ml Base Oil
- ✓ 60 ml Vinegar
- ✓ 2 200-ml clean bottles, New or Recycled
- ✓ 1 100-ml Bottle, New or Recycled
- ✓ 1 200 ml Spray Bottle, New or Recycled
- ✓ 1 500 ml Bottle, New or Recycled

1. NATURAL SHAMPOO

Ratio: 30 drops Essential Oil : 200 ml Liquid Soap

200 ml Bottle
200 ml Liquid Soap Mix (see Soap for recipe)
30 drops Essential Oils as below

Blend Suggestions

dr = drops

Everyday Use for Normal Hair
10 dr Lavender, 8 dr Chamomile, 6 dr Lemon, 6 dr Geranium

Oily Hair
10 dr Geranium, 8 dr Chamomile, 6 dr Lavender, 6 dr Tea Tree

Dry Hair
10 dr Chamomile, 8 drops Lemon, 6 dr Geranium, 6 dr Lavender

Damaged
10 dr Chamomile, 10 dr Geranium, 5 dr Tea Tree, 5 dr Lavender

Dandruff
10 dr Tea Tree, 8 dr Chamomile, 6 dr Lavender, 6 dr Lemon

This recipe gives you a base for all your shampoo blends. For babies and children up to 2 years, halve the quantity of essential oils.

If you don't wish to make your own shampoo base, buy a natural baby shampoo with no added aromas. You will not get as much foam when you wash with this shampoo since there is no foaming agent added (it's not needed), so don't worry. Your hair is getting clean just the same.

Mix: Pour Liquid Soap Mix into bottle; add to this your Essential Oils and shake well.

2. NATURAL CONDITIONER

Ratio: 3 ml Essential Oil : 47ml Base Oil: 150 ml Water

200 ml Bottle
47 ml Base Oil
1 cup Boiled (Hot) Water
20 drops (1 ml) Chamomile Essential Oils

Massage into hair and leave for 2-3 minutes. Rinse off. This recipe gives you a base for all your conditioner blends. If you don't wish to make your own conditioner base, buy a natural gentle conditioner (baby conditioner) with no added aromas.

Mix: To hot water, add Essential Oil and then add Base Oil mix. Shake well thoroughly. This product will need to be shaken before each use as no dispersant was added. (A dispersant is a chemical to stop the ingredients from separating. A quick shake does the same thing.)

Babies

Using Essential Oils for babies is beneficial because the properties work on their bodies and their mind, giving them great memories of aromas. Combine this with touching and massage, and your baby will thrive emotionally and physically.

Oils for Babies and Toddlers
Newborn – Chamomile, Geranium, Lavender
2-6 months – Chamomile, Geranium, Lavender and Eucalyptus
6-12 months – Chamomile, Geranium, Lavender, Neroli, Tea tree and Eucalyptus

3. HOT OIL TREATMENT

Ratio: 20 drops Essential Oil : 100 ml Base Oil

100 ml Bottle
10 drops Lemon
99 ml Base Oil

Pour approximately a tablespoon (2 tablespoons for long hair) into a small bowl and heat in microwave or double boiler until warm (not boiling). Pour into palm and massage through hair. Add another tablespoon if required to give a nice coverage over hair.

Wrap hair in plastic wrap (or plastic bag, or shower cap) and then wrap a towel around. This will keep the heat in, giving extra benefit to your treatment.

Allow to remain on hair for 20-30 minutes. Rinse out and style as usual. If you find your hair is still too oily, you may shampoo and condition your hair.

Mix: To give your hair a lovely revitalizing treatment, blend the Base Oil with the Essential Oils and shake thoroughly.

4. LEAVE-IN CONDITIONER

Ratio: 50 ml Conditioner : 150 ml Water

200 ml Spray bottle
50 ml Conditioner (with Essential Oils added)
150 ml Boiled (Cooled) Water

Shake well and spray into hair on a daily basis to manage frizz and fly-away hair

Mix: Combine conditioner and water and shake well. Spray onto wet hair and style as needed or spray onto dry hair to refresh and renew.

5. SHINE RINSE

Ratio: 60 ml Vinegar : 440 ml Water

500 ml Bottle
60 ml Vinegar
440 ml Boiled (Cooled) Water

Use this after shampoo and before conditioner to help remove build-up from previous chemical-based products. It will enhance your color and vitality of your hair. It may take up to two weeks after you first start using natural products to really see the benefit of this rinse because it slowly removes all build-up and chemical and product residue from your hair.

Mix: Mix Essential Oils, Vinegar and Water into bottle and shake well. Apply to hair and leave for 2-3 minutes. Rinse out thoroughly.

RECIPES: A-Z OF HAIR CARE

ALOE VERA GEL

Ratio: 10 drops Essential Oil : 200 ml Aloe Vera Gel

200 ml Jar
200 ml Aloe Vera Gel
10 drops Lavender Essential Oil

Aloe Vera Gel is similar to commercial hair gels but it is not as sticky when dried; it still holds well. When rinsed out, it leaves hair soft and manageable.

Mix: Mix together Aloe Vera Gel and Essential Oils; the gel will get foggy in color. Apply gel to palm of hand and work through the same as commercial hair gel.

CLEANSER

Ratio: ½ cup Bicarb : 250 ml Water

250 ml Jar
1 cup Warm Water
½ cup of Bicarb

This cleanser is ideal after using large quantities of products in your hair such as for special occasion hair styles.

Mix: Combine Bicarb and Water. Apply to hair and massage through gently. Leave in for 2-3 minutes and rinse thoroughly. Shampoo and condition as usual.

CONDITIONERS
Hair needs to be conditioned after shampooing to balance the ph and moisturize the hair

NATURAL CONDITIONER

Ratio: 3 ml Essential Oil : 47ml Base Oil : 150 ml Water

200 ml Bottle
47 ml Base Oil
1 cup Boiled (Hot) Water
20 drops Chamomile Essential Oils

Massage into hair and leave in for 2-3 minutes before rinsing out.

This recipe gives you a base for all your conditioner blends. If you don't wish to make your own conditioner base, buy a natural gentle conditioner (baby conditioner) with no added aromas.

Mix: To hot water, add Essential Oil and then Base Oil. Mix together (shake well) thoroughly. The ingredients in this mix may separate, because no dispersant was used. (A dispersant is a chemical to stop the ingredients from separating.) Before use, shake well to remix ingredients.

EGGY CONDITIONER

Ratio: 20 drops Essential Oil : 5ml Base Oil : 1 Egg Yolk : 190 ml Water

200 ml Bottle
20 drops Chamomile Essential Oils
5 ml Base Oil
1 Egg Yolk
190 ml Boiled (Cooled) Water

This recipe gives you a base for all your conditioner blends. If you don't wish to make your own conditioner base, buy a natural gentle conditioner with no added aromas.

Mix: Beat egg yolk until it forms soft peaks. Fold in oil and beat again. Pour in water and slowly mix together. Pour into bottle, add Essential Oils, and shake well. The ingredients in this mix may separate, because no dispersant was used. (A dispersant is a chemical to stop the ingredients from separating.) Before use, shake well to remix ingredients.

Massage into hair and leave in for 2-3 minutes before rinsing out.

DARK HAIR BRIGHTENER

Ratio: 10 drops Essential Oil : 200 ml Water

200 ml Bottle
200 ml Boiled (Cooled) *Water*
8 drops Chamomile Essential Oil
2 drops Geranium Essential Oils

Use this blend to add extra shine and bring out the highlights of dark hair.

Mix: Add Essential Oils to water and shake well. Pour over hair after conditioning as final rinse. Do not rinse out.

FAIR HAIR BRIGHTENER

Ratio: 10 drops Essential Oil : 200 ml Water

200 ml Bottle
200 ml Boiled (Cooled) *Water*
8 drops Lemon Essential Oil
2 drops Geranium Essential Oils

Use this to add extra shine and bring out the highlights of fair hair.

Mix: Add Essential Oils to water and shake well. Pour over hair after conditioning as final rinse. Do not rinse out.

FRIZZ AWAY TREATMENT

Ratio: 10 drops Essential Oil : 200 ml Aloe Vera Gel

200 ml Jar
4 tablespoons Natural Yogurt or Natural Body Lotion
1 Egg
6 drops Chamomile Essential Oil

This treatment is ideal for taming frizzy hair and still leaves hair bouncy and shinny.

Mix: Blend together all ingredients and store in air tight container in refrigerator. Pour over hair after shampooing and rinse with cool water (not warm). No need to use conditioner. Style as usual.

HAIR GEL

Ratio: 6 drops Essential Oil : 1 teaspoon Gelatin: 250 ml Water

250 ml Jar
1 cup Boiling Water
1 teaspoon Gelatin
6 drops Chamomile Essential Oil

Mix: Add gelatin to boiling water and stir until dissolved. Add in Essential Oils and stir again. Allow to set and stir before use. Keep refrigerated. Apply gel to palm of hand and work through the same as commercial hair gel.

HAIR SPRAY

Ratio: 10 drops Essential Oil : Lemon: Orange: 500 ml Water

250 ml Bottle
1 Lemon
1 Orange
2 cups Boiling Water
10 drops Chamomile Essential Oil

This is a natural hairspray that is chemical free and smells divine.

Mix: Cut lemon and orange into pieces and add to saucepan along with water. Boil and reduce by half. Allow to cool, and then strain into spray bottle. Add essential oils. Store in refrigerator. This will last about 7-10 days. (Add 2 tablespoons of Vodka and the mix will last in the refrigerator for about one month.)

HEAD LICE

Head lice and nits are unfortunately a part of school children's life. They attach themselves to the strains of hair and live off the scalp. There are two different issues when treating head lice. First, the lice themselves need to be killed and removed; second, the nits or eggs need to be removed. Head lice lay eggs at the bottom of the hair shaft and can be hard to get off. The best way to get them off is combing with a special head lice comb (the metal comb is a lot more effective than the plastic) and conditioner, Essential Oil and Base Oil mix. This is an effective solution because the oil helps the eggs slip off and the conditioner and Essential Oils stun the head lice which can be removed from hair with comb.

HEAD LICE SHAMPOO

Ratio: 20 drops Essential Oil : 200 ml Liquid Soap Mix

200 ml Bottle
200 ml Liquid Soap Mix
20 drops Essential Oil as below

Use this first to kill the head lice, ideal for large infestations as first step in process.

Mix 1: Geranium 10 drops, Lavender 4 drops, Tea Tree 4 drops, Tea Tree 2 drops

Mix 2: Geranium 25 drops, Lavender 15 drops

Pour Liquid Soap Mix into bottle, add Essential Oils, and shake well. Apply to hair as you would normal shampoo; massage though, especially onto scalp and base of hair. Rinse out and treat with Head Lice Treatment

HEAD LICE HAIR TREATMENT

Ratio: 40 drops Essential Oil : 30 Base Oil : 170 ml Natural Conditioner

200 ml Bottle
170 ml Natural Conditioner
30 ml Base Oil
40 drops Essential Oil as below

Mix 1: Geranium 10 drops, Lavender 4 drops, Tea Tree 4 drops, Tea Tree 2 drops

Mix 2: Geranium 25 drops, Lavender 15 drops

Mix: Pour conditioner into bottle. (If you need this quickly and have no natural conditioner made up, use the cheapest bottle of conditioner from supermarket since it will be in the hair for about 20 minutes.) Add Base Oil and Essential Oils and shake well. Apply to hair and leave for 10 minutes. Do not remove. Place towel around the neck and divide the hair up into small sections. Comb through, wiping conditioner onto tissues after each comb. (This will contain lice and eggs and you don't want to return it to hair.) Continue until all hair is completed.

This will need to be done again before 7 days and then again 7 days later to break the breeding cycle since any eggs left may hatch and the process starts again.

HEAD LICE DAILY SPRAY

Ratio: 10 drops Essential Oil : 20 ml Base Oil : 40 ml Natural Conditioner : 140 ml Water

200 ml Bottle
40 ml Natural Conditioner
20 ml Base Oil
140 ml Boiled (Cooled) *Water*
10 drops Essential Oil as below

Mix 1: Eucalyptus 6 drops, Tea Tree 4 drops

Mix 2: Geranium 6 drops, Lavender 4 drops

Pour conditioner, Base Oil and water into bottle. Shake well. Add Essential Oils and shake again

Use this spray each day to help prevent head lice. Alternate Mix 1 and Mix 2 because the lice get used to a product. This help make the hair uninviting to them.

HOT OIL TREATMENT

Ratio: 20 drops Essential Oil : 100 ml Base Oil

100 ml Bottle
10 drops Lemon
99 ml Base Oil

Pour approximately a tablespoon (2 tablespoons for long hair) into small bowl and heat in microwave or double boiler until warm (not boiling). Pour into palm and massage through hair. Add another tablespoon if required to give a nice coverage over hair.

Wrap hair in plastic wrap (or plastic bag, or shower cap) and then wrap a towel around. This will keep the heat in, giving extra benefit to your treatment.

Allow to remain on hair for 20-30 minutes. Rinse out and style as usual. If you find your hair is still too oily, you may shampoo and condition your hair.

Mix: To give your hair a lovely revitalizing treatment, blend the Base Oil with the Essential Oils and shake thoroughly.

LEAVE-IN CONDITIONER

Ratio: 50 ml conditioner: 150 ml Water

200 ml Spray bottle
50 ml Conditioner (with Essential Oils added)
150 ml Boiled (Cooled) Water

Shake well and spray into hair on a daily basis to manage frizz and fly-away hair

Mix: Combine conditioner and water and shake well. Spray onto wet hair and style as needed or spray onto dry hair to refresh and renew.

MOUSSE, EGGY

Ratio: 6 drops Essential Oil : 4 Egg Whites

200 ml Jar
4 egg whites
6 drops Chamomile Essential Oil

Separate egg whites into bowl and beat until soft peaks form. Fold in Essential Oils and store in air-tight container in refrigerator. Apply to hair as you would commercial hair mousse.

PSORIASIS HAIR TREATMENT

Ratio: 20 drops Essential Oil : 200 ml Base Oil : 200 ml Bottle

8 drops Tea Tree Essential Oil
6 drops Chamomile Essential Oil
6 drops Lavender Essential Oil
200 ml Base Oil

This treatment may assist in the healing of psoriasis and relieve some of the symptoms associated with it. Pour approximately a tablespoon (2 tablespoons for long hair) into a small bowl and heat in microwave or double boiler until warm (not boiling). Pour into palm and massage through hair. Add another tablespoon if required to give a nice coverage over hair.

Wrap hair in plastic wrap (or plastic bag, or shower cap) and then wrap a towel around. This will keep the heat in, giving extra benefit to your treatment.

Allow to remain on hair for 20-30 minutes. Rinse out and style as usual. If you find your hair is still too oily, you may shampoo and condition your hair.

Mix: Blend the Base Oil with the Essential Oils and shake thoroughly.

SHAMPOOS

NATURAL SHAMPOO

Ratio: 30 drops Essential Oil : 200 ml Liquid Soap

200 ml Bottle
200 ml Liquid Soap Mix (see Soap for recipe)
30 drops Essential Oils as below

Blend Suggestions

dr = drops
Everyday Use for Normal Hair
10 dr Lavender, 8 dr Chamomile, 6 dr Lemon, 6 dr Geranium

Oily Hair
10 dr Geranium, 8 dr Chamomile, 6 dr Lavender, 6 dr Tea Tree

Dry Hair
10 dr Chamomile, 8 drops Lemon, 6 dr Geranium, 6 dr Lavender

Damaged
10 dr Chamomile, 10 dr Geranium, 5 dr Tea Tree, 5 dr Lavender

Dandruff
10 dr Tea Tree, 8 dr Chamomile, 6 dr Lavender, 6 dr Lemon

This recipe gives you a base for all your shampoo blends. For babies and children up to 2 years, halve the quantity of essential oils.

If you don't wish to make your own shampoo base, buy a natural baby shampoo with no added aromas. You will not get as much foam when you wash with this shampoo since there is no foaming agent added (it's not needed), so don't worry. Your hair is getting clean just the same.

Mix: Pour Liquid Soap Mix into bottle; add to this your Essential Oils and shake well.

– Hair Care Help–

EGGY SHAMPOO

Ratio: 1 Egg : 20 drops Essential Oil : 50 ml Liquid Soap : 100 ml Water

200 ml Bottle
1 Egg, mix as below
20 drops Essential Oil as below
100 ml Warm Water
50 ml Liquid Soap or Shampoo Mix

Blend Suggestions

 dr = drops

Everyday Use for Normal Hair
10 dr Lavender, 8 dr Chamomile, 6 dr Lemon, 6 dr Geranium

Oily Hair
10 dr Geranium, 8 dr Chamomile, 6 dr Lavender, 6 dr Tea Tree

Dry Hair
10 drops Chamomile, 8 drops Lemon, 6 dr Geranium, 6 dr Lavender

Damaged
10 dr Chamomile, 10 dr Geranium, 5 dr Tea Tree, 5 dr Lavender

Dandruff
10 dr Tea Tree, 8 dr Chamomile, 6 dr Lavender, 6 dr Lemon

Mix: Whisk together all ingredients and pour into bottle. Keep refrigerated. Wet hair and use to wash hair as normal. Rinse thoroughly; follow with Build-up Rinse (if required) and conditioner. Pat dry and style.

SHINE RINSE

Ratio: 60 ml Vinegar : 440 ml Water

500 ml Bottle
60 ml Vinegar
440 ml Boiled (Cooled) Water

Use this after shampoo and before conditioner to help remove build-up from previous chemical-based products. It will enhance your color and vitality of your hair. It may take up to two weeks after you first start using natural products to really see the benefit of this rinse because it slowly removes all build-up and chemical and product residue from your hair.

Mix: Mix Essential Oils, Vinegar and Water into bottle and shake well. Apply to hair and leave for 2-3 minutes. Rinse out thoroughly.

STRAIGHTENING HAIR SPRAY

Ratio: 10 drops Essential Oil : 250 ml milk

250 ml Spray Bottle
250 ml Milk
10 drops Chamomile Essential Oil

Help straighten your hair without harsh chemicals. Use the protein in milk to relax the hair and allow it to straighten. Hair becomes shiny and silky and will not smell of rancid milk (only leave on as directed). It can be dried with a hair dryer or naturally.

Mix: Pour milk into Spray Bottle, add Essential Oils, and shake well. Spray hair with mixture until saturated. Leave on for one hour and shampoo and condition as usual.

SECTION 10

Perfume Pampering

I love the clear scents you get when you blend pure Essential Oils together and create your own perfumes. I love that you can create your own fragrances as well as complimentary products to give you an aromatic feeling of being pampered and perfumed.

Years ago when I first learned about perfumes I discovered that Essential Oils are the basis of most fragrances, with the high quality perfumes being made from many different Essential Oils all blended together to create a symphony of fragrance.

We all know that expensive perfumes seem to last and the aromas are nicer on your senses. Did you know that these quality fragrances are made from Essential Oils?

By creating your own, you have the benefits of the more expensive perfumes; you create a perfume that holds its fragrance and releases its notes gradually over a period of time.

Cheaper perfumes have none of these properties because they are made from fragrance oil or low quality synthetic oils. This is why you need to apply them more frequently and the fragrance doesn't have the depth of the more expensive perfumes.

If you want to take your perfume to the next level and create an exquisite layering system, you will find that your skin will love the pampering and you will delight in how beautiful and luxurious you feel. Your friends will assume you are now wearing an expensive perfume but it will only cost you a small amount compared to the high quality perfumes.

A while back I create a layering system for a friend of mine, which was simple to make and wonderful to wear. Together we had already created a perfume that she loved, but I wondered if I could create a layer of perfume for her using only natural products instead of the chemical-base products that irritated her skin.

Would Essential Oils be able to linger and perform over the day? I know how the notes of Essential Oils work, (see in Chapter 1 "Essential Oil Notes"), but we wanted the same lingering aromas you get from a high quality perfume range. Was it possible with Essential Oils or was this function created using chemical additives?

With a bit of trial and error (wasn't too hard and lots of fun), I created my first (of many) perfume layering ranges. You can image my friend's joy when she used these products; she was surprised and delighted at the results and even more delighted when we worked out the cost to make them. She now has several perfumes she likes and she makes herself a layering range when she is into a perfume—different ones for different times of the year, day or night or depending on what mood she is in.

I am not as diligent as my friend. I use my layers some days, but other days I use a quick spray or dab of perfume on the way out the door, but that still uplifts me.

To create your own perfumes and layering system you need to first create your own perfume; then if you wish you can pamper yourself and create your own layering system, which is definitely worth your time/

Remember that even commercial perfumes smell different on different people because everyone's body heats up at different rates. The perfume releases its notes at different times. So try your perfume on your skin and allow the Essential Oil molecules to be released and appreciated. If your friends love your perfume, get them to try it on before whipping some up for them. An extra drop of one Essential Oil may make smell even better on your friend's skin.

THE BENEFITS OF YOUR OWN PERFUME BLENDS

The benefits of creating your own perfumes are that they are totally yours and can show your individual personality. Making your own perfumes gives you the highest quality products at a fraction of the cost, without compromising on quality and fragrance.

This chapter will allow you to create your own products and give you a basic understanding of creating your own blends. The blends I suggests are just that: suggestions. Please enjoy the fun of experimenting.

PERFUMERY'S ESSENTIAL 5

This is the only section where adding additional oils is necessary. For perfumes, the notes of the Essential Oils are important and you need to have oils from top, middle and base. This is not as important in the other sections as their properties and uses outweigh the note values.

A perfume is started with a base note such as Ylang Ylang as it fixes the perfume; then the other notes are built onto its notes.

Next is added our middle note, Jasmine with its sweet warm heady aroma. (It is an expensive oil, so if you don't want to purchase such as expensive oil or if the headiness of it is too strong, you can use Palmarosa and Geranium. Use half of each for blend for a rose-like fragrance.)

This is followed by another middle (and top) note. Lavender, a wonderful oil for perfumes, is a bridging oil that brings blends together. This is completed with our top note. You can use Lemon, an invigorating citrus; Geranium, with sweet floral aromas and a slight minty overtone; and Chamomile, with its fruity sweet and fresh aroma.

Because not everyone likes floral perfumes, I have also given other alternatives. The blends are given with 10-drop amounts, which you can multiply to suit your recipe. For example, to make a perfume you need 80 drops. You would multiply this by eight for cologne. All of this is explained with the recipes.

When creating your own perfumes, first decide on your base note and build from there. Add your middle notes second and then add your top notes to finish the blend.

PERFUME AND THEIR AROMATIC NOTES

As you can see, only your imagination and your nose (olfactory gland) will limit your choices of Essential Oils for Perfumery.

When creating your own, make up a 10-drop blend in 1 ml Base Oil. If you want to experiment remember that Jojoba is expensive so use cheaper base oil for test blends. Remember you must blend with Base Oil before putting it on your skin as neat Essential Oils are too strong for topical applications; they must be diluted.

Ratio: 10 drops Essential Oil : 1 ml Base Oil

Add base notes oils first, followed by middle, and completed with top note Essential Oils.

Here are some of the more common Essential Oils and their notes.

TOP NOTES	MIDDLE NOTES	BASE NOTES
* *denotes Top and Middle note or Middle and Base Note*		
Basil	Black Pepper	Cedarwood
Bergamot	Chamomile	Cinnamon *M-B
Citronella	Clary Sage* T-M	Clove
Eucalyptus	Cypress	Frankincense
Grapefruit	Geranium	Ginger
Lemon	Ginger	Myrrh
Lime	Jasmine	Patchouli
Neroli* T-M	Lavender * M-T	Rose
Orange	Marjoram	Sandalwood
Peppermint	Palmarosa	Vetiver
Sage	Petitgrain	Ylang Ylang
Rosemary *T-M	Pine	
	Tree Tea* T-M	
	Thyme	

THE COST COMPARISON OF YOUR PERFUME STARTER KIT

When you first purchase high quality, 100-percent pure Essential Oils, you may think that you have spent a lot of money for such a small quality of oils, but a little goes a long way.

The cost may still seem high when making perfumes but compare it to high quality perfumes and you will definitely save money and create a fragrance unique to you.

Essential Oils from a 12 ml bottle will provide you with 240 drops of Essential Oil. Compare the cost of buying the six products.

I have priced these products on cheapest available (perfume products that use essential oils, quality not fragrance oils). Remember that you can pick up cheap perfumes for around $5-10, but they don't last. Furthermore, you have to reapply them more regularly and you don't get that high quality aroma you get with amazing perfumes.

Purchased Products (Generic or Cheapest Product Available)	Cost	Products Created Using Essential 5 Essential Oils and Household Products	Cost
Perfume Soap	$9.95	Perfume Soap	$1.30
Body Oil – 100 ml	$29.95	Body Oil – 100 ml	$15.00
Perfumed Talc – 200 g	$15.95	Perfumed Talc – 200 g	$1.50
Eau de Cologne – 100 ml	$39.95	Eau de Cologne – 100 ml	$20.00
Deodorant – 100 ml	$29.95	Deodorant – 100 ml	$10.00
Perfume – 10 ml	$49.95	Perfume – 10 ml	$11.00
TOTAL COST	**$175.70**	**TOTAL COST**	**$58.80**

Perfumery Layering System

Imagine creating a complete system of aromas. You will feel pampered and be delighted with how complete your fragrance feels and lingers.

Soap, Liquid Soap, or Bath Oil
Wash and clean your body with your aromatic product

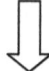

Body Lotion, Body Oil, or Bath Oil
Apply to (or massage) your entire body with Body Lotion or have a luxurious bath with the Bath Oil

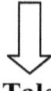

Talc
Gently pat dry your skin and talc it

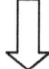

Eau de Toilette or Eau de Cologne
Add your Eau de Toilette or Cologne to your body.
A gentle spray is all that is required

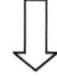

Deodorant
Now that you body is truly fragrant, add your deodorant to help eliminate unpleasant body odors.

Perfume or Perfume Oil
Complete your aromatic experience with your Perfume or Perfume Oil. Dab onto pulse points, wrists, neck throat—even behind the knees and ankles and between your breasts. Remember use only one drop as this is a highly concentrated product.

PERFUME BLEND USING ESSENTIAL 4 OILS

These blends are formulated in 10-drop blends so multiply to create blends. For example, perfume needs 80 drops (dr) so you multiply the blend by 8.

DREAM	FLORAL LOVE	JAZZY JASMINE	CITRUS FLOWER
3 dr Lavender	4 dr Lavender	2 dr Lavender	2 dr Lavender
3 dr Jasmine	3 dr Jasmine	5 dr Jasmine	2 dr Jasmine
2 dr Ylang Ylang	2 dr Ylang Ylang	2 dr Ylang Ylang	2 dr Ylang Ylang
2 dr Geranium	1 dr Chamomile	1 dr Geranium	4 dr Lemon
SENSUAL BLISS	**FRUITY FUN**	**FLORAL ZING**	**TRANQUILITY**
1 dr Lavender	2 dr Lavender	3 dr Lavender	2 dr Lavender
3 dr Jasmine	2 dr Jasmine	2 dr Jasmine	3 dr Chamomile
4 dr Ylang Ylang	3 dr Ylang Ylang	2 dr Ylang Ylang	3 dr Ylang Ylang
2 dr Geranium	3 dr Lemon	3 dr Geranium	2 dr Geranium

USING OTHER ESSENTIAL OILS TO CREATE MORE PERFUME RANGES

Perfumes are such individual choices so if you would prefer a blend without a floral base, here are some other ideas for you to try.

These blends are formulated in 10-drop blends so multiply to create blends. For example, perfume needs 80 drops so you multiply the blend by 8.

FLORAL BEAUTY	CITRUS	CHI	ORIENTAL
2 dr Lavender	1 dr Bergamot	2 dr Orange	2 dr Lemon
2 dr Rosemary	2 dr Lemon	1 dr Lavender	2 dr Lavender
3 dr Jasmine	3 dr Sandalwood	3 dr Cypress	3 dr Patchouli
3 dr Ylang Ylang	4 dr Patchouli	4 dr Cedarwood	3 dr Sandalwood
SENSUAL	EXOTIC	SPICY	FRESH
2 dr Lavender	2 dr Bergamot	1 dr Rose	2 dr Orange
1 dr Jasmine	2 dr Rose	2 dr Patchouli	2 dr Jasmine
3 dr Ylang Ylang	2 dr Jasmine	3 dr Sandalwood	3 dr Vetiver
4 dr Patchouli	4 dr Cedarwood	4 dr Vetiver	3 dr Sandalwood
SPICY FRUIT	GODDESS	PRINCESS	EXOTIC SPICY
2 dr Cinnamon	3 dr Bergamot	3 dr Coriander	3 dr Jasmine
3 dr Lime	2 dr Palmarosa	1 dr Frankincense	3 dr Neroli
4 dr Rose	3 dr Rose	3 dr Juniper	4 dr Orange
5 dr Ylang Ylang	4 dr Sandalwood	4 dr Orange	
GREEN FRESH	FLORAL FRUITY	FLORAL SPICY	HEAVENLY
2 dr Bergamot	3 dr Neroli	2 dr Cinnamon	1 dr Lavender
3 dr Ylang Ylang	2 dr Mandarin	3 dr Lime	3 dr Bergamot
4 dr Jasmine	3 dr Ylang Ylang	2 dr Geranium	2 dr Jasmine
1 dr Patchouli	2 dr Vanilla /Vetivert	3 dr Ylang Ylang	3 dr Sandalwood
DAISY	LAVENDER LOVE	MACHO MAN	SPICY MAN
2 dr Lavender	3 dr Lavender	2 dr Lemon	2 dr Bergamot
2 dr Bergamot	2 dr Lemon	2 dr Rosewood	2 dr Basil
3 dr Rosewood	3 dr Palmarosa	3 dr Cedarwood	2 dr Lavender
3 dr Patchouli	1 dr Vetiver	3 dr Sandalwood	4 dr Pettigraine

RECIPES: PERFUME STARTER KIT

Ingredients List

You will need the following items to create one complete kit:

- ✓ Lavender Essential Oil
- ✓ Geranium Essential Oil
- ✓ Chamomile Essential Oil
- ✓ Lemon Essential Oil
- ✓ Jasmine Essential Oil
- ✓ Ylang Ylang Essential Oil
- ✓ 1 15-ml Clean Glass Bottle, New or Recycled
- ✓ 2 100-ml Clean Glass Spray Bottles, New or Recycled
- ✓ 1 100-ml Clean Glass Bottle, New or Recycled
- ✓ 1 200-ml Clean Glass Bottle, New or Recycled
- ✓ 1 Clean Large Salt Shaker or Jar with Holes in Lid
- ✓ Jelly Mold or Container to Form Soap
- ✓ ½-bar Soap
- ✓ 130.5 ml Vodka (or Pure Alcohol)
- ✓ 195 ml Base Oil
- ✓ 100 ml Vinegar
- ✓ 150 grams Corn Starch
- ✓ 50 gram Bicarb
- ✓ 1 teaspoon Glycerin

Create the complete kit or just your favorite perfume product.

1. PERFUMED SOAP

Ratio: 10 drops Essential Oil : Bar Soap: 1tablespoon Base Oil

Soap Mold or Jelly Mold
1 bar Pure Soap
10 drops Essential Oil (of your blend)
1 tablespoon Base Oil

Create your own perfume soap by melting down a natural bar. Although you can buy soap-making ingredients and make it from scratch, that means a lot more initial expense and time. If you love making soaps, then this may be another option.

Mix: Place grated soap and water into a microwave safe bowl (or use double boiler for stove) and cook on high for 1-2 minutes. We want only to soft it; we don't want to turn it into liquid.

When soft add Essential Oils and 1 tablespoon Base Oil. Mix thoroughly and press into mold. If using a jelly mold or small container, line with greaseproof or plastic wrap to enable you to remove the soap. Allow to set, creating a fragranced soap bar.

2. PERFUMED BODY OIL

Ratio: 100 drops (5 ml) Essential Oil : 95 Base Oil

100 ml Glass Bottle
100 drops (5 ml) Essential Oils (Your Blend)
95 ml Base Oils

The recipe gives you very high moisturizing oil. Use this if you prefer to use body oil instead of a moisturizer cream. The Body Oil will give the skin a supple appearance and is ideal for dry skin or skin in harsh climates where even the loveliest of skin has a tendency to dry up. Apply all over body, or apply directly after your bath when your skin is still damp. Gently pat dry.

3. TALC

Ratio: 10 drops Essential Oil : 150gr Cornstarch: 50gr Bicarb

200 ml Jar (Large Salt Shaker or Talc Bottle)
10 drops Essential Oils (Your Blend)
150 gram Cornstarch
50 gram Bicarb

Talc is great for your body; the Bicarb extends the blend and gives its deodorizing benefits and when talc is combined with cornstarch, it feels wonderful and luxurious.

Mix: Blend together dry ingredients and slowly drop Essentials into mix. Stir thoroughly after each drop. Pour into shaker or into large container, and use powder puff to apply.

4. EAU DE COLOGNE

Ratio: 120 drops (6ml) Essential Oils : 70 ml Vodka: 24ml Water

100 ml Dark Glass Spray Bottle
120 drops (6 ml) Essential Oils (Your Blend)
60 ml Vodka
24 ml Water

Eau de Cologne is ideal as part of your layering system. It is used as a spray and is about 12 percent concentrate of your perfume blend; it also adds a further dimension of layering.

Mix: Mix together the Essential Oils and Vodka, stirring the mixture slowly to disperse all the Essential Oil droplets. Allow the mixture to stand for 2-3 days (in a cool dark place) and then add water. Allow the mixture to stand for another 2-3 days (in a cool dark place), and then you may use it. You can make and use it straightaway, but for a better product this time line is important. If you would like to create a deeper product, allow the complete product to stand for six weeks in a cool dark area to allow the oils to mature.

5. DEODORANT

Ratio: 60 drops Essential Oil : 1 teaspoon Glycerin : 100 Vinegar : 97 ml Base Oil

200 ml Spray Bottle
100 ml Vinegar
97 ml Base Oil
60 drops (3 ml) Essential Oils (Your Blend)
1 teaspoon Glycerin

The sweat glands of the feet and armpits are different from anywhere else on the body. Vinegar is a natural deodorant because it dries up the older perspiration (odor-causing) and allows the armpits to remain dry and fresh. When combined with Essential Oils and Base Oils, the solution will provide good aroma and keep moisturizing arms pits, preventing dry skin.

Mix: Combine all ingredients and shake well. Let it stand for 3-4 days and shake gently before each use.

6. PERFUME

Ratio: 80 ml (4 ml) drops Essential Oil : 10.5 ml Alcohol: ½ ml Water

15 ml Dark Glass Bottle
4 ml Essential Oils (Your Blend)
10.5 ml Vodka
½ ml Water

This perfume can be the *pièce de résistance* of your layering system or your "splash on and run out the door perfume." Your own perfume is a created blend that is totally yours.

Remember this is a very concentrated blend and a little will go a long way.

Mix: Mix together the Essential Oils and Vodka, stirring the mixture slowly to disperse all the Essential Oil droplets. Allow the mixture to stand for 2-3 days (in a cool dark place) and then add water. Allow the mixture to stand for another 2-3 days (in a cool dark place), and then you may use it. You can make and use it straightaway, but for a better product this time line is important. If you would like to create a deeper product, allow the complete product to stand for six weeks in a cool dark area to allow the oils to mature.

RECIPES: A-Z OF PERFUMERY PRODUCTS

BATH OIL

200 ml Bottle
100 ml (5ml) Essential Oils (Your Blend)
30 ml Base Oil
160 ml Vodka

Love oil and baths and the way it gives moisture to your skin and relaxes you but don't like the oil ring after? How about bath oil without the oil ring?

This blend will nearly dissolve completely in the bath water. A little goes a long way so don't go overboard. Add to your bath, a great start to your perfume layering system.

Mix: Mix together the Essential Oils and Vodka, stirring the mixture slowly to disperse all the Essential Oil droplets. Allow the mixture to stand for 2-3 days (in a cool dark place) and then add water. Allow the mixture to stand for another 2-3 days (in a cool dark place), and then you may use it. You can make and use it straightaway, but for a better product this time line is important. If you would like to create a deeper product, allow the complete product to stand for six weeks in a cool dark area to allow the oils to mature.

BODY OIL

Ratio: 100 drops (5 ml) Essential Oil : 95 Base Oil

100 ml Glass Bottle
100 drops (5 ml) Essential Oils (Your Blend)
95 ml Base Oils

The recipe gives you very high moisturizing oil. Use this if you prefer to use body oil instead of a moisturizer cream. The Body Oil will give the skin a supple appearance and is ideal for dry skin or skin in harsh climates where even the loveliest of skin has a tendency to dry up. Apply all over body, or apply directly after your bath when your skin is still damp. Gently pat dry.

DEODORANT

Ratio: 60 drops Essential Oil : 1 teaspoon glycerin: 100 Vinegar: 97 ml Base Oil

200 ml Spray Bottle
100 ml Vinegar
97 ml Base Oil
60 drops (3 ml) Essential Oils (Your Blend)
1 teaspoon Glycerin

The sweat glands of the feet and armpits are different from anywhere else on the body. Vinegar is a natural deodorant because it dries up the older perspiration (odor-causing) and allows the armpits to remain dry and fresh. When combined with Essential Oils and Base Oils, the solution will provide good aroma and keep moisturizing arms pits, preventing dry skin.

Mix: Combine all ingredients and shake well. Let it stand for 3-4 days and shake gently before each use.

EAU DE COLOGNE

Ratio: 120 drops (6ml) Essential Oils : 70 ml Vodka: 24ml Water

100 ml Dark Glass Spray Bottle
120 drops (6 ml) Essential Oils (Your Blend)
60 ml Vodka
24 ml Water

Eau de Cologne is ideal as part of your layering system. It is used as a spray and is about 12 percent concentrate of your perfume blend; it also adds a further dimension of layering.

Mix: Mix together the Essential Oils and Vodka, stirring the mixture slowly to disperse all the Essential Oil droplets. Allow the mixture to stand for 2-3 days (in a cool dark place) and then add water. Allow the mixture to stand for another 2-3 days (in a cool dark place), and then you may use it. You can make and use it straightaway, but for a better product this time line is important. If you would like to create a deeper product, allow the complete product to stand for six weeks in a cool dark area to allow the oils to mature.

EAU DE TOILETTE

Ratio: 60 drops (4ml) Essential Oils : 60 ml Vodka : 36ml Water

100 ml Dark Glass Spray Bottle
3 ml Essential Oils (Your Blend)
60 ml Vodka
36 ml Water

Eau de Toilette is ideal as part of your layering system and can be used use as a spray. It is about 6 percent concentrate of your perfume blend adding a further dimension of layering. It is lighter than the Eau de Cologne and the choice of usage is purely individual.

Eau de toilette is ideal as part of your layering system or for a lighter scent.

Mix: Mix together the Essential Oils and Vodka, stirring the mixture slowly to disperse all the Essential Oil droplets. Allow the mixture to stand for 2-3 days (in a cool dark place) and then add water. Allow the mixture to stand for another 2-3 days (in a cool dark place), and then you may use it. You can make and use it straightaway, but for a better product this time line is important. If you would like to create a deeper product, allow the complete product to stand for six weeks in a cool dark area to allow the oils to mature.

LIQUID SOAP

500 ml Bottle (Pump or Squirt Bottle is best)
50 drops (2.5 ml) Essential Oils (Your Blend)
½ bar Natural Soap
500 ml Water

I love the smoothness of a liquid soap and the kids love using it also.

Mix: Grate a half bar of soap and add to 500 ml Water. Place broken up soap (or grated) into a saucepan or microwave-proof dish with water and bring to boil. Boil until the soap has become a slurry; this should take approximately 10-15 minutes. Allow to cool until just warm and pour into blender. (Do not put hot ingredients into blender.) Blend until smooth and pour into a bottle. Store and use for all recipes requiring soap.

PERFUME OIL

25 ml Dark Glass Bottle
20 drops (1 ml) Essential Oils (Your Blend)
9 ml Base Oil

If you like your perfume as an oil, this blend is for you. It is richer than the perfume and doesn't contain any alcohol. Also it ideal for more sensitive skins.

Mix: Blend together Essential Oils and Base Oils. Shake gently to mix together. Dab onto pulse points.

PERFUME

Ratio: 80 ml (4 ml) drops Essential Oil : 10.5 ml Alcohol : ½ ml Water

15 ml Dark Glass Bottle
4 ml Essential Oils (Your Blend)
10.5 ml Vodka
½ ml Water

This perfume can be the *pièce de résistance* of your layering system or your "splash on and run out the door perfume." Your own perfume is a created blend that is totally yours.

Remember this is a very concentrated blend and a little will go a long way.

Mix: Mix together the Essential Oils and Vodka, stirring the mixture slowly to disperse all the Essential Oil droplets. Allow the mixture to stand for 2-3 days (in a cool dark place) and then add water. Allow the mixture to stand for another 2-3 days (in a cool dark place), and then you may use it. You can make and use it straightaway, but for a better product this time line is important. If you would like to create a deeper product, allow the complete product to stand for six weeks in a cool dark area to allow the oils to mature.

SOAP

Ratio: 10 drops Essential Oil : Bar Soap: 1 tablespoon Base Oil

Soap Mold or Jelly Mold
1 bar Pure Soap
10 drops Essential Oil (of your blend)
1 tablespoon Base Oil

Create your own perfume soap by melting down a natural bar. Although you can buy soap-making ingredients and make it from scratch, that means a lot more initial expense and time. If you love making soaps, then this may be another option.

Mix: Place grated soap and water into a microwave safe bowl (or use double boiler for stove) and cook on high for 1-2 minutes. We want only to soft it; we don't want to turn it into liquid.

When soft add Essential Oils and 1 tablespoon Base Oil. Mix thoroughly and press into mold. If using a jelly mold or small container, line with greaseproof or plastic wrap to enable you to remove the soap. Allow to set, creating a fragranced soap bar.

SPLASH COLOGNE

100 ml Glass Bottle
40 drops (2 ml) Essential Oils (Your Blend)
80 ml Vodka
18 ml Water

Splash this on for a refreshing aroma

Mix: Mix together the Essential Oils and Vodka. Stir the mixture slowly to disperse all the Essential Oil droplets. Allow the mixture to stand for 2-3 days (in a cool dark place) and then add water. Allow the mixture for another 2-3 days (in a cool dark place) then you may use it.

TALC

Ratio: 10 drops Essential Oil : 150gr Cornstarch: 50gr Bicarb

200 ml Jar (Large Salt Shaker or Talc Bottle)
10 drops Essential Oils (Your Blend)
150 gram Cornstarch
50 gram Bicarb

Talc is great for your body; the Bicarb extends the blend and gives its deodorizing benefits and when talc is combined with cornstarch, it feels wonderful and luxurious.

Mix: Blend together dry ingredients and slowly drop Essentials into mix. Stir thoroughly after each drop. Pour into shaker or into large container, and use powder puff to apply.

SECTION 11

Gorgeous Gift Ideas

LOVE GIVING GIFTS THAT DELIGHT

Do you love giving gifts? Do you love giving high quality gifts that you know they will love?

I love giving gifts and usually try to get something that my friends and family will use and appreciate. Sometimes this is hard especially if they are the sort of person who really has everything they need.

I have found over the years that people receive handmade gifts exceptionally well. In this day and age when you can buy just about anything you want and people have more and more "stuff," people appreciate a beautiful handmade gift that they can see you have taken time and effort to make.

The other benefit of making gifts from Essential Oils is even though the gifts are handmade, they can look and will feel expensive and high quality. I remember giving bath salts once and the person was quite happy about it, but a couple of days later I got a phone call saying how wonderful the bath salts were to use compared to other products she had used in the past and could she have more. I gave her the recipe.

For that added touch, always present your gifts elegantly in boxes and packaging (keep it simple).

A-Z OF GIFT IDEAS

BATH BOMBS

160 grams Bicarb
40 gram of Citric Acid
20 drops Essential Oil (Your Blend)
1 tablespoon Base Oil
1 teaspoon Food Coloring, Herbs, or Flower Petals for Coloring

Combine the natural fizz of Bicarb that stimulates your mind and body with the wonderful properties of pure Essential Oils to create bath bombs. Bath bombs will help the body and mind and are fun for the whole family

Mix: Combine all dried ingredients in a bowl add Essential Oils 5 drops at a time and mix extremely well and then add Base Oil. If required, add more Base Oil. Your mixture should hold together into a basic shape. Press mixture into mold and allow to set for 2-3 hours. Press out and store in air tight container.

Uses
Baths, Foot Baths

BATH OIL

200 ml Bottle
100 ml (5ml) Essential Oils (Your Blend)
195 ml Base Oil

Enjoy the luxury of bathing with oil and the way it gives moisture to your skin and relaxes you? Use warm water to relax and hotter water to stimulate.

Mix: Pour Base Oil into bottle and add Essential Oil blend. Mix thoroughly and use.

BATH OIL - Dissolving

200 ml Bottle
100 ml (5ml) Essential Oils (Your Blend)
30 ml Base Oil
160 ml Vodka

200 ml Bottle
100 ml (5ml) Essential Oils (Your Blend)
30 ml Base Oil
160 ml Vodka

Love oil and baths and the way it gives moisture to your skin and relaxes you but don't like the oil ring after? How about bath oil without the oil ring?

This blend will nearly dissolve completely in the bath water. A little goes a long way so don't go overboard. Add to your bath, and enjoy the aromas for relaxations and stress relief.

Mix: Mix together the Essential Oils and Vodka, stirring the mixture slowly to disperse all the Essential Oil droplets. Allow the mixture to stand for 2-3 days in a cool dark place. Then add water. Allow the mixture to stand for another 2-3 days in a cool dark place. Then you may use it. While you can make it in all one go, you'll make for a better product if you follow this time line.

BATH SALTS

200 grams Epsom Salts
20 drops Essential Oil (Your Blend)
1 tablespoon Bicarb
1 teaspoon Food coloring, herbs, or flower petals for coloring

Combine the properties of these truly amazing natural products to create a simple and effective bath product. Add your Essential Oils depending on your mood and desires and let your troubles float away.

Mix: To the Epsom Salts, stir in Bicarb and coloring product (if required). Mix well. Then add Essential Oil blend and mix again.

Place in a clear jar; tie with a ribbon and label. This will delight your friends.

– Gorgeous Gift Ideas –

BODY OIL

100 ml Glass (or Plastic) Bottle
100 drops (5 ml) Essential Oils (Your Blend)
95 ml Base Oils

Wrap and present! It's as easy as that. Body Oils of this quality are truly gorgeous gift ideas. This recipe gives you a wonderful oil product.

Use this if you prefer to use body oil instead of a moisturizer cream. The Body Oil will give the skin a supple appearance and is ideal for dry skin or skin in harsh climates where even the loveliest of skin has a tendency to dry up. Apply all over body, or apply directly after your bath when your skin is still damp. Gently pat dry.

Mix: Pour Base Oil into bottle and add Essential Oils. Mix well.

Uses
Moisturizing, Massage, Showering, Room Spray (Add 2 tablespoons to water and shake well.)

FACE SPRAY

20 ml glass Atomizer Bottle
10 drops Lemon Essential Oils
5 drops Lavender Essential Oil
5 drops Chamomile Essential Oil
2 drops Geranium Essential Oil
1 ml Base Oil
13 ml Water

This is a wonderful little gift and, if presented in a beautiful atomizer, will be truly welcomed. A refreshing face spray freshens your senses and sooths your mind. It allows you to absorb the oils quickly at home or take your face spray in your purse and use it at time of daily stress.

Mix: Combine Essential Oils, Base Oil and Water in atomizer and shake gently to combine all ingredients. Shake before each use as there is no dispersant (usually chemical based) in this blend to keep the oils and water from separating.

LAVENDER SACHETS

2 Small Squares of Cloth (8 cm square)
Needle and thread to sew into pillows
Dried Lavender or Cotton Wool
10 drops Lavender Essential Oil

Sachets are deal for airing cupboards and linen drawers.

Sew together two piece of cloth (wrong side out) on three sides and turn in to form a pillow. Fill with dried Lavender or cotton wool and drop in Essential Oil. Sew up last side. Add a bow for a complete look.

PAPER MÂCHÉ GIFTS

Using Paper Mâché to Create Gift Products

How to Make Paper Mâché
Flour
Water
Newspaper, any recyclable paper

Paper mâché is the art of sticking paper together with flour and water (makes glue) in layers to foam a shape..

Mix: Mix together 1 part flour to 2 parts water until you get the consistency of a thick glue (slightly runny – not like a paste). Mix well and remove all lumps. If you live in a high humidity area, then add 3 tablespoons of salt to prevent mold.

SCENTED BEAD

Paper mâché mix
1 drop Lavender Essential Oil per Bead (change oil to suit)

Scented beads are ideal for display on tables or placed in drawers to fragrance clothes.

Roll paper mâché into ball shapes, adding one drop of Essential Oil to each ball. Make ball about 2 cm diameter and place on greaseproof paper to dry. When dry, paint color of your choice and present in beautiful box or bowl.

SCENTED MOBILES

Paper mâché Mix
1 drop Lavender Essential Oil per Shape
1 drop Chamomile Essential Oil per Alternative Shape

Create a mobile infused with Lavender and Chamomile to help babies sleep. As the mobile moves in the breeze, it will release the aromas.

Form paper mâché into shapes adding one drop of Essential Oil to each shape. To make shapes you can use molds and press the paper mâché into it. Place on greaseproof paper to dry. When dry, pierce a piece of wire through top to make a loop to hang mobile. Paint with the colors of your choice. Use a coat hanger (or heavy wire to give structure to mobile) to hang shapes.

SCENTED PENDANTS

Paper mâché Mix
1 drop Lavender Essential Oil per Shape (change oil to suit)

Imagine creating a heart pendant and infusing it with oil, or creating a star or moon infused with Chamomile for calmness. Use your imagination. You will love coming up with new uses.

Form paper mâché into ball shapes, adding one drop of Essential Oil to each ball. Make shape suitable size of pendant and place on greaseproof paper to dry. When dry, pierce the top and hang on a cord or a chain necklace in the color of your choice. Present it in beautiful box.

SCENTED DRINK COASTERS

Paper mâché Mix
2 drops Lemon Essential Oil per Coaster (change oil to suit)

These drink coasters are a fabulous gift idea. When someone puts a hot drink on a coater, the heat will warm it up and release the fragrance.

Form paper mâché into a coaster shape, adding two drop of Essential Oil to each shape. An egg ring is the ideal shape for a coaster; make it as thick or thin as you like. Place on greaseproof paper to dry. When dry, paint the color of your choice and present it in beautiful box.

PLAY DOUGH

2 cups of Plain Flour
4 tablespoons of Cream Of Tartar
2 tablespoons of Cooking Oil
1 cup of Salt
2 cups of Boiling Water
Food Coloring

Mix 1:
10 drops Lavender Essential Oil
10 drops Chamomile Essential Oil
5 drops Geranium

Mix 2:
10 drops Lemon Essential Oil
8 drops Geranium Essential Oil
5 drops Lavender Essential Oil
2 drops Chamomile Essential Oil

Create scented play dough as gifts for children. It encourages them to play and allows them to correlate aromas with pleasant activities. Using Mix 1 prior to rest time can allow the mind to associate these oils with resting and sleeping. The Mix 2 blend can be used to calm restless and hype children

Mix: Mix all ingredients (except Food Coloring) into bowl and microwave for 5 minutes. Stir and fold out onto floured board and knead well. Add more flour until a smooth Play Dough-consistency. Break up into balls if you want more than one color and add a teaspoon of food coloring at a time until you are happy with the color, kneading as you go to blend color. Add Essential Oils and knead well. Present in an air tight container or zip lock bags.

SECTION 12

Aromatherapy

WHAT IS AROMATHERAPY

Aromatherapy is a healing therapy that utilizes the properties and aromas of essential plant oils. It is the application and inhalation of Essential Oils from aromatic plants. Aromatherapy uses pure Essential Oils skillfully and in a controlled manner to influence mind, body, and soul for physical and emotional health and well being.

The basic principle of Aromatherapy is to strengthen the self-healing processes by indirect stimulation of the immune system. This can range from deep and penetrating therapeutic uses to extreme subtlety of a unique fragrance; the depth of pure Essential Oils is unending.

We are using the benefits of Aromatherapy without being aware; we perfume our bodies. We use smells around the house for to eliminate odor and provide a scent. We use sage, rosemary, and lemon in the food. Pure Essential Oils gives us the very best quality and the convenience of a concentrated product for many applications.

Aromatherapy is already in our lives. Everyone has emotional responses whether pleasant or unpleasant to certain scents. Using Aromatherapy is a way to improve the quality of life on a physical, emotional, and spiritual level.

Essential Oils can easily and effectively be used in your own skin care preparations, for health and vitality, and for general wellness.

In today's society most household goods are chemical-based. The air we breathe, the food we eat, the products we use contain more chemicals than we would like. The cumulative effect of these and the unknown effects as they react with us on a daily basis cannot be good for us anymore than the chemical overload is for the planet.

Alternatives need to be found. Right under own noses are nature's precious miracles and delights of creation, pure essential oils.

Clinical research has shown that an environment on which disease, virus, fungus, bacteria etc cannot live may be created using essential oils. This involves using "pure" Essential Oils and treatments that many believe have a chemical effect of the body.

The fragrance of a plant is the Essential Oil in its natural form. A number of complex bio-chemicals including antibiotics, antiseptics, and vitamins in their natural state are part of the Essential Oils.

AROMATHERAPY HISTORY

Dating back thousands of years is the use of plants, aromas and natural ingredients for healing and improving health. Ancient civilizations of Egypt, China, the Middle East, India, and Greece have used essential oils.

Hippocrates, the father of medicine, said that "the way to health is to have an aromatic bath and scented massage every day." He recognized that burning certain aromatic substances offered protection against contagious diseases.

In Egypt, exotic perfumes were used in abundance by pharaohs and their families for offerings to the gods and as embalming essential oils. Bath houses used by the Greeks and Romans were famous for using aromatic oils.

In the Middle East plants were widely used for medicinal and therapeutic properties. Essential Oils were brought to Europe by the crusaders and developed during the Middle Ages into one of the most sought after forms of natural healing.

In the tenth century AD an Arabian alchemist discovered the method of distillation. Rose was the first oil extracted this way. From this, rosewater became a popular scent and even found its way to Europe during the Crusades.

The word *aromatherapy* was coined in the 1920s by French perfumer Rene Gattefosse. When he badly burnt his hand and arm, he reacted by immersing it in neat Lavender Essential Oil and found that it healed very rapidly without infection or apparent scarring. He then went on the research the properties of pure Essential Oils and found that Lavender and many others oils were antiseptic and better than the chemical antiseptics available at the time. His research led him to writing *Aromatherapie* in 1928.

An Austrian biochemist, Marguerite Maury is also recognized as an important figure in the pioneering of the modern approach to aromatherapy. Even though her main interest was skin care, she understood the overall healing potential of Essential Oils. Marguerite Maury set up in London the first aromatherapy clinic. Essential Oils are currently used in pharmaceutical preparations.

> **Did You Know?**
> Aromatherapy is already in our lives. Everyone has emotional responses, whether pleasant or unpleasant, to certain scents. A memory of a fragrance can trigger emotions.

HOW ESSENTIAL OILS ARE MADE

Referred to as the plant "life force," Essential Oils occur widely in the plant kingdom. They are the minute droplets of liquid occurring in glands; hairs or veins of flowers, leaves, back, wood, and resin roots; or fruit peel of a plant.

Essential Oils are made several ways

Steam distillation. (Chamomile, Lavender, Geranium) The plant is placed on a grid inside a distillation vat and steam is passed through under pressure. The heat causes the cell walls of the plant to break down releasing the Essential Oil as a vapor. The vapor is passed through cooling tanks, where it condenses. The steam and oil vapors are cooled and separated; as a result most Essential Oils are lighter than water.

Expression. (Citrus Oils) The peel of a citrus fruit has oil glands containing globules of essential oils. They are squeezed from the peel after the pulp has been separated.

Extraction. (Rose, Jasmine, Orange Flower) Extraction is mainly used for more delicate flowers.

ESSENTIAL OIL PROPERTIES

Most of the Essential Oils have healing properties, and some have many properties allowing them to be used in a variety of recipes. These are some of the Essential Oils I have used over the years and the ones I have found to be most commonly used and recognized.

TOP NOTES	MIDDLE NOTES	BASE NOTES
* *denotes Top and Middle note or Middle and Base Note*		
Basil	Black Pepper	Cedarwood
Bergamot	Chamomile	Cinnamon *M-B
Citronella	Clary Sage* T-M	Clove
Eucalyptus	Cypress	Frankincense
Grapefruit	Geranium	Ginger
Lemon	Ginger	Myrrh
Lime	Jasmine	Patchouli
Neroli* T-M	Lavender * M-T	Rose
Orange	Marjoram	Sandalwood
Peppermint	Palmarosa	Vetiver
Sage	Petitgrain	Ylang Ylang
Rosemary *T-M	Pine	
	Tree Tea* T-M	
	Thyme	

A-Z ESSENTIAL OILS

BASIL
Note: Top

This refreshing and inspiring oil helps improve energy. It helps clears the sinuses, stimulates circulation, and promotes digestion, especially in the respiratory system. It encourages clear thinking and decision making. Basil assists with warming of joints to relieve symptoms of stiffness and swelling. It is useful for insect bites, acne, and general skin irritations because of its antiseptic qualities.

Botanical Name: *Ocimum basilicum*
Plant Part: Leaves and flowers
Extraction: Steam distilled
Origin: Italy
Strength of Aroma: Strong

Blends Well with: Bergamot, Clary Sage, Clove, Eucalyptus, Lemon, Neroli, and Rosemary

Aromatic Scent: Clear, herbaceous, and light; refreshing with a faint balsamic woody back note and a lasting sweetness

History: In Greek its name means "royal remedy" or "'king." In Mediterranean countries, India, and Asia, the culinary plant is used extensively in cooking.

<u>**Cautions:**</u> Avoid during pregnancy.

BERGAMOT

Note: Top

Uplifting with its deliciously fresh and invigorating citrus aroma, Bergamot is also useful for oily and blemished skin as a skin conditioner. It is a very effective antidepressant and a great oil to use at the start of the day. It is useful in cleaning cuts and grazes and assisting with minor skin infections.

Botanical Name: *Citrus bergamia*
Plant Part: Crude fruit peel
Extraction Method: Cold press
Origin: Italy
Strength of Aroma: Medium

Blends Well with: Black Pepper, Clary Sage, Cypress, Frankincense, Geranium, Jasmine, Lavender, Mandarin, Nutmeg, Orange, Rosemary, Sandalwood, Vetivert, and Ylang Ylang

Aromatic Scent: The aroma of the Essential Oil is basically citrus, yet it is fruity and sweet with a warm spicy floral quality, reminiscent of Neroli and Lavender oil.

History: The name *Bergamot* is derived from the city Bergamo in Lombardy where the oil was first sold. It is also found in the Ivory Coast, Morocco, Tunisia, and Algeria.

Cautions: Bergamot oil can cause severe burns when used on sensitive skin that has been exposed to sunlight.

BLACK PEPPER

Note: Middle

Black Pepper is useful in the treatment of muscular pain, stiffness, poor circulation, and muscle tone. The warm energizing oil is used to promote mental clarity and combat tiredness,

Botanical Name: *Piper nigrum*
Plant Part: Dried berries
Extraction Method: Steam distillation
Origin: India
Strength of Aroma: Medium

Blends Well with: Ginger, Eucalyptus, Frankincense, Marjoram, Basil, Rosemary, Lime, Jasmine, and Bergamot

Aromatic Scent: Fresh and warm with a spicy aroma

History: Pepper was moving from India over 4,000 years ago. It has always been a key component of the spice trade.

Cautions: Avoid during pregnancy

CEDARWOOD
Note: Base

Cedarwood is considered an aphrodisiac with grounding and inspiring qualities and is used for acne, arthritis, bronchitis, coughing, cystitis, dandruff, dermatitis, stress. It is warming, uplifting, and toning as well as comforting and reviving. Used in the deterrent of moths and part of an antiseptic spray, it is also helpful for long standing complaints such as arthritis, chest infections, and acne.

Botanical Name: *Cedrus atlantica*
Plant Part: Wood extraction
Method: Steam distillation
Origin: USA
Strength of Aroma: Medium to Strong

Blends Well with: Citrus Oils, Rosemary, Chamomile, Eucalyptus, and many more

Aromatic Scent: Cedarwood Atlas has a woody, sweet smell, reminiscent of artificial mothballs or balsamic.

History: This Cedarwood originates in the Atlas Mountains in North Africa. In former times, linen chests were frequently crafted from this wood to keep moths out. To date, clothes hangers are frequently crafted from this wood. The ancient Egyptians used to embalm, for cosmetics and perfumery.

Uses: Drop onto cotton wool balls to deter moths. Drop onto hangers for clothes storage. Get as part of an antiseptic spray.

Cautions: Avoid during pregnancy.

CHAMOMILE

Note: Middle

Chamomile is gentle enough for babies and children and works very well with Lavender. Chamomile has a long tradition in herbal medicine. The flowers were used in many cures including an herbal tea to cure insomnia. The Essential Oil is useful in the treatment of aches and pains in muscles and joints. Treatment of symptoms of PMS with Chamomile is also beneficial especially when the symptoms are related to stress.

Botanical Name: *Chamaemelum nobile*
Plant Part: Flower head
Extraction Method: Steam distilled
Origin: Italy
Strength of Aroma: Strong

Blends Well with: Geranium, Lavender, Rose, Neroli, Marjoram, Cedarwood, Frankincense, Rosewood, Clary Sage, and Ylang Ylang.

Aromatic Scent: The relaxing aroma of this essential oil, sometimes described as like "apples and straw," is exotic and rich.

History: This herb has been used for medicinal purposes and skin therapy for a long time, in particular in Europe. In ancient Egypt it was considered sacred and dedicated to the sun-god Ra. Chamomile has been used throughout history by the Arabic doctors and the Saxons; in the Victorian times, it was used along with Lavender to calm hysteria.

CINNAMON
Note: Middle

Cinnamon is a very powerful oil that should be used in small doses. It helps to relieve tension and daily stress and generally warm limbs and assist with circulation and muscular aches and pains.

Botanical Name: *Cinnamonum zeylanicum*
Plant Part: Bud, leaf and tree
Extraction Method: Distilled
Origin: Indonesia
Strength of Aroma: Medium

Blends Well with: Ginger, Grapefruit, Lavender, Rose, Neroli, , Frankincense, Rosemary, Clary Sage, and Ylang Ylang.

Aromatic Scent: A sweet spicy scent with slight musky undertone. The aroma is synonymous with hot donuts

History: Cinnamon was part of the spice trade between Indian, China and Egyptians dating back of 4,000 years.

Cautions: Avoid during pregnancy.

CITRONELLA
Note: Top

Citronella is credited with having therapeutic properties as an antiseptic, deodorant, insecticide, parasitic, and stimulant. Most people will still associate it as an insecticide. Many commercial repellents contain it, and it's often used in combination with Cedarwood to produce a pleasant smelling natural insect repellent.

Botanical Name: *Cymbopogon nardus*
Plant Part: Gum
Extraction Method: Steam
Origin: Sri Lanka
Strength of Aroma: Strong

Blends Well with: Bergamot, Orange, Cedarwood, Geranium, Lemon, Orange, Lavender, and Pine

Aromatic Scent: A well-rounded lemon citrus scent, though it is much softer than actual Lemon. It also has subtle wood tone.

History: Citronella Ceylon Essential Oil was one of the world's dominant insect repellents before the introduction of DEET. Recent history has indicated that Citronella is once again becoming the product of choice for health conscious customers.

Cautions: Citronella may irritate sensitive skin.

CLARY SAGE
Note: Middle

Clary Sage is viewed as an antidepressant, antispasmodic, deodorant, sedative and tonic. It is well known for providing a euphoric feeling and assisting with depression and cleansing greasy hair.

Botanical Name: *Salvia sclarea*
Plant Part: Leaves and flowers
Extraction Method: Steam
Origin: Bulgaria
Strength of Aroma: Medium to Strong

Blends Well with: Bergamot, Cedarwood, Roman and German Chamomile, Geranium, Jasmine, Lavender, Neroli, Orange, Rosewood, Sandalwood, and Ylang Ylang

Aromatic Scent: Clary Sage Essential Oil has an earthy, fruity, and floral aroma that is both nutty and herbaceous.

History: The name *Clary Sage* is derived from the Latin word for "clear," probably because the herb was once used for clearing mucous from the eyes. During the sixteenth century it was also used as a replacement for hops for brewing beer in England.

CLOVE
Note: Base

Clove Bud Essential Oil is an effective agent for minor pains and aches (particularly dental pain) and is helpful when battling flu and colds. It is a powerful antiseptic.

Botanical Name: *Syzgium aromaticum*
Plant Part: Buds
Extraction Method: Steam
Origin: India
Strength of Aroma: Medium to Strong

Blends Well with: other spice oils, Citronella, Grapefruit, Lemon, Orange, Peppermint, Rosemary, and Rose

Aromatic Scent: spicy and rich like actual cloves.

History: The word clove comes from the Latin word *clavus*, meaning nail, since the shaft and head of the clove bud resemble a nail. Cloves and nutmeg were among the most precious of items of Europe of the 16th and 17th centuries, and they were worth more than their weight in gold.

Cautions: Clove Bud Oil can cause sensitivity in some and should be used in diluted form. It should also be avoided during pregnancy.

CYPRESS
Note: Middle

Used as a bereavement oil to encourage a sense of comfort, Cypress is also good for oily skin and hair and excessive perspiration. It may be helpful for stress-related states and nervous exhaustion.

Botanical Name: *Cupressus sempervirens*
Plant Part: Leaves/cones and trees
Extraction Method: Distillation
Origin: Mediterranean countries
Strength of Aroma: Medium

Blends Well with: Bergamot, Juniper, Lavender, Lemon, Rosemary, Orange, and Sandalwood

Aromatic Scent: Similar to pine with woody refreshing aroma with smoky overtones.

History: The Ancient Greeks burned this in ceremonies and the tree was dedicated to Hades, Greek god of the Underworld. They are grown around graveyards and churches because of their growth pattern (tall and skinny); they are symbolically pointing to heaven.

Cautions: Avoid during pregnancy; may change or regulate menstrual cycles.

EUCALYUPTUS
Note: Top

Eucalyptus has attracted much popularity for giving relief from cold and flu. The refreshingly sweet scent of Eucalyptus Essential Oil is enjoyed by many for its pleasant aroma and easy assimilation. It is a great chest rub and antiseptic and ideal for cleansing and relief of itches. This is a truly an amazing Essential Oil that relieves the itchiness of insect bites. Antiseptic qualities make it suitable for cleaning.

Botanical Name: *Eucalyptus radiata*
Plant Part: Leaves
Extraction Method: Steam
Origin: China
Strength of Aroma: Strong

Blends Well with: Pine, Thyme, Lavender, Rosemary, marjoram, Cedarwood, and Lemon

Aromatic Scent: Eucalyptus has a very herbaceous scent. It also has soft wood undertones.

History: Eucalyptus Essential Oil has long been used in homes in Australia. In Spain, the timber of Eucalyptus was used in construction. The earliest research into the properties of Eucalyptus was carried out in 1870 by Doctor Cloez.

FRANKINCENSE
Note: Base

Frankincense is a warm, spicy oil suitable in treating anxiety. Used traditionally for meditation and relaxation, it helps in easing colds, flu, sinusitis and hay fever; and assists with the rejuvenation of aging skin. As a skin tonic, it is effective with sores, carbuncles, wounds, scars, and skin inflammation.

Botanical Name: *Boswellia rivae*
Plant Part: Resin
Extraction Method: CO_2
Origin: Africa
Strength of Aroma: Strong

Blends Well with: Basil, Bergamot, Cardamom, Cedarwood, Chamomile, Cinnamon, Clary Sage, Coriander, Geranium, and Ginger Essential Oils

Aromatic Scent: Frankincense has a woody, spicy, haunting smell. It is slightly camphoric but is regarded as more pleasant.

History: Frankincense is from the French word *Franc* meaning "luxuriant" or it could be "real incense." Also known as Olibanum, Frankincense was used by the ancient Egyptians as an offering to the gods and as a rejuvenating facemask.

GERANIUM
Note: Middle

Geranium has therapeutic properties as an astringent, diuretic, antiseptic, anti-depressant, tonic, antibiotic, anti-spasmodic and as an anti-infectious agent. It aids against travel sickness and assists with irritations associated with dermatitis, eczema, and psoriasis.

Botanical Name: *Pelargonium graveolens*
Plant Part: Herb
Extraction Method: Steam distillation
Origin: Egypt
Strength of Aroma: Strong

Blends Well with: Basil, Bergamot, and Carrot seed, Cedarwood, Citronella, Clary Sage, Grapefruit, Jasmine, Lavender, Lime, Neroli, Orange, and Rosemary

Aromatic Scent: A scent that is both sweet and herbaceous while carrying some subtle notes similar in character to Rose.

History: The plants originated from South Africa as well as Reunion, Madagascar, Egypt and Morocco. In the 17th century European countries such as Italy, Spain and France, it was planted around the house to help keep evil spirits away.

Cautions: Avoid during pregnancy.

GINGER
Note: Middle / Base

Ginger is known for its assistance with colds and flu, nausea, muscle aches, circulation issues and arthritic pain. It also has warming properties that help to combat loneliness, and depression. Ginger is also viewed as an aphrodisiac based on its energizing properties.

Botanical Name: *Zingiber officinale*
Plant Part: Root
Extraction Method: Steam
Origin: France
Strength of Aroma: Medium to Strong

Blends Well with: Bergamot, Sandalwood, Ylang-Ylang, and other spice oils

Aromatic Scent: Warm, spicy, woody scent with a hint of lemon and pepper.

History: The plant is said to originate from India, China and Java, but it is also native to Africa and the West Indies. It is believed that Ginger was brought to Europe between the 10th and 15th century as both a condiment and spice. It has been used for medicinal purposes since the ancient times. It is mentioned in literature from the Greeks, Romans, and Arabians.

GRAPEFRUIT
Note: Top

Grapefruit is thought to be a spiritual up-lifter, and able to ease muscle fatigue and stiffness. It can purify congested, oily, and acne-prone skin; it is also useful as a cleanser for skin and hair and helps prevent dandruff.

Botanical Name: *Citrus paradisi*
Plant Part: Crude peel
Extraction Method: Cold press
Origin: France
Strength of Aroma: Medium

Blends Well with: Other members of the Citrus family, Rosemary, Cypress, Lavender, Geranium, and generally most spice oils

Aromatic Scent: Grapefruit Pink Essential Oil has a fresh, tart citrus smell that is very characteristic of the fruit.

History: The differences between the White and Pink Grapefruit are minor. The difference in cost is simply an example of supply and demand; there is more pink grapefruit produced because it is sweeter than the white variety.

JASMINE
Note: Middle

The highly fragrant aromas of Jasmine are known for their aphrodisiac qualities and for assisting in calming, working as a sedative, and reducing of stress. It helps skin retain its elasticity and softness and assists with the lightening of stretch marks when combined with Lavender. It is one of the most expensive Essential Oil and many synthetic copies have been created. It must be an Essential Oil to receive the therapeutic benefits. Because of the high price of Jasmine, alternative and less expensive oils could be used just as effectively.

Botanical Name: *Jasminum officinate*
Plant Part: Flowers/tree
Extraction Method: Effleurage
Origin: Egypt, France, Italy, Morocco
Strength of Aroma: Strong

Blends Well with: Bergamot, Frankincense, Lavender, Geranium, Rose, Palmarosa, Sandalwood, Orange, and Ylang Ylang

Aromatic Scent: Sweet, warm, flowery aroma, slightly heady

History: Native to Persia and Kashmir, this oil has long been used in love potions because it is reputed to have aphrodisiac properties. Jasmine is found in over 80 percent of women's fragrances and 30 percent of men's fragrances.

Cautions: Do not use during pregnancy as it inhibits the flow of milk.

JUNIPER OR JUNIPER BERRY
Note: Middle

Juniper Berry is valued for its detoxifying properties. Juniper is used to bolster the spirits and strengthen and stimulate the nerves. It can assist in the treatment of arthritis, acne, dermatitis, psoriasis, and cellulite. It is also used for antiseptic, skin cleanser, and insect bites.

Botanical Name: *Juniperus communis*
Plant Part: Leaves
Extraction Method: Steam distilled
Country of Origin: India
Strength of Aroma: Medium to strong

Blends Well with: Bergamot, Cypress, Frankincense, Geranium, Orange, Grapefruit, Sandalwood, and Rosemary

Aromatic Scent: Clear refreshing with woody overtones (slightly peppery).

History: Juniper was used by the Ancient Egyptians and Greeks to ward off infections and as part of the embalming process. They also used juniper berries for a variety of medical purposes including flatulence and indigestion; it was considered able to restore lost youth.

Cautions: Do not use during pregnancy as it may affect menstruation. Replace with sandalwood.

LAVENDER
Note: Top / Middle

If you were only going to have one Essential Oil, then this is the one. Lavender is an affordable oil with many healing properties.

Lavender's distinctive but light floral aroma is one of the most recognized and it can be credited in the revival of aromatherapy and using essential oils.

This oil is one of the few that can be used directly onto skin (neat) as a topical application on burns and sunburn. It is an antiseptic, and it can be used for sleep assistance and relaxation. Suitable for use in burners and diffusers because of its clean, floral aromas, it alleviates anxiety, tension, and stress. Plus it is excellent for relaxation blends: lavender blends well with most oils, especially citrus and floral.

Botanical Name: *Lavandula angustifolia*
Plant Part: Flower head
Extraction Method: Steam distilled
Origin: France
Strength of Aroma: Strong
Blends Well with: Bay, Bergamot, Chamomile, Citronella, Clarysage, Geranium, Jasmine, Lemon, Mandarin, Orange, Palmarosa, Patchouli, Pine, Tangerine, Thyme, Rosemary, Rosewood, and Ylang Ylang

Aromatic Scent: A sweet floral note preferred by many

History: It is believed that the Romans and the Benedictine monks introduced it to rest of Europe. The Romans dropped lavender flower heads in the communal baths and part of their antiseptic blends. Medieval herbalists recommended using it for head lice and prevention of bed bugs.

LEMON
Note: Top

Lemon is prized for its high anti-bacterial properties. On skin and hair it can be used for its cleansing effect as well as for its antiseptic properties. It is refreshing and cooling and may assist with the ability to concentrate.

Botanical Name: *Citrus limon*
Plant Part: Peel of the fruit
Extraction Method: Cold pressed
Origin: Italy
Strength of Aroma: Strong

Blends Well with: Lavender, Chamomile, Frankincense, Eucalyptus, Ginger, Juniper, Neroli, Ylang Ylang, and Sandalwood

Aromatic Scent: Similar to fresh lemon rinds except richer and more concentrated

History: The fruit was well-known in Europe by the Middle Ages, and Greeks and Romans were advocates of its therapeutic properties. Lemon Essential Oil reached the height of its fame when the British began using the citrus fruit to counteract the effects of scurvy.

LIME
Note: Middle

Lime is a refreshing, relaxing oil that soothes anxiety, stress, and nervous tension. As with most citrus, it is has excellent cleansing properties and may assist in removal of excess oils from skin.

Botanical Name: *Citrus aurantifolia*
Plant Part: Peel and fruit
Extraction: Distillation
Origin: Italy and West Indies
Strength of Aroma: Medium

Blends Well with: Bergamot, Basil, Geranium, Lavender, Neroli, Rose, and Rosemary

Aromatic Scent: Zesty with sharp fruit fresh undertones

History: Discovered as prevention to scurvy, it was added to the 18th century naval ships.

Cautions: Avoid use if you spend long periods in the sunlight; may irritate sensitive skin

MARJORAM
Note: Middle

Marjoram is a fabulous oil to sooth the nerves and calm the mind. It is a warming oil that helps relieve muscular pain and joint swelling, It provides relief from stomach cramps, heart burn and chest congestion. Marjoram is helpful in blends for the elderly.

Botanical Name: *Origanum marjorana*
Plant Part: Leaves/flowering heads/herb
Extraction Method: Distillation
Origin: Egypt, Spain and Morocco
Strength of Aroma: Medium

Blends Well with: Bergamot, Cedarwood, cypress, Clary Sage, Lavender, Orange, Rosemary, and Ylang Ylang

Aromatic Scent: Warm spicy and penetrating with herbaceous notes

History: Recorded use can be found back in the Ancient Greek times with the women putting it on their head as a relaxant and possibly to relieve migraines. The goddess Aphrodite is reputed to have regarded it a s symbol of happiness.

Cautions: Do not use during pregnancy.

MYRRH
Note: Base

Myrrh is a calming oil that provides relief from coughs and bronchial irritation. It has been known to be used for meditation and stress relief. It helps the skin retain softness and suppleness and benefits aging skin.

Botanical Name: *Commiphora myrrha*
Plant Part: Stem, branches, gum resin
Extraction: Steam distillation
Origin: Southeast Arabia and North Africa
Strength of Aroma: Strong

Blends Well with: Frankincense Lavender, Lemon, Patchouli, and Sandalwood

Aromatic Scent: Balsamic and musky with smoky notes

History: Ancient Egyptians used myrrh for mummification as well as medication.

Cautions: Do not use during pregnancy.

ORANGE
Note: Top

Orange is helpful as an antidepressant, antiseptic, antispasmodic, aphrodisiac, carminative, cordial, deodorant, digestive, and stimulant (nervous), tonic (cardiac, circulatory). It has also been applied to combat colds, constipation, dull skin, flatulence, the flu, gums, slow digestion, and stress.

Botanical Name: *Citrus sinensis*
Plant Part: Fruit/peel
Extraction Method: Expression
Origin: Mediterranean
Strength of Aroma: Medium to strong

Blends Well with: Frankincense, Cypress, Ginger, Geranium, Jasmine, Lavender, Petitgrain, and Rose

Aromatic Scent: Sweet Orange oil has a sweet, citrus smell much like the orange peels it is derived from, only more intense and concentrated.

History: It is native to China, but it is believed that Sweet Orange was brought to Europe by the Arabs in the first century along with the Bitter Orange.

Cautions: Avoid if exposure to the sun may occur; may irritate young or sensitive skin

PALMAROSA
Note: Middle

The Palmarosa's properties include uses as an antiseptic, bactericidal, digestive, stimulant, and tonic. It is used extensively as a fragrance component in cosmetics, perfumes, and especially soaps because of its excellent tenacity and its action against viral illnesses and bacteria – coupled with the attractive smell. As a result, it is a great oil to use to disinfect a room. Its properties assist with water retention and moisturizing and it stimulates cell regenerations.

Botanical Name: *Cymbopogon martinii*
Plant Part: Grass
Extraction Method: Steam
Origin: India
Strength of Aroma: Medium to strong

Blends Well with: Bergamot, Jasmine, Sandalwood, Ylang Ylang Petitgrain, Geranium, Rosewood, Sandalwood, and Cedarwood

Aromatic Scent: Palmarosa Essential Oil has a sweet, floral fragrance with a hint of rose.

History: Palmarosa was known as Indian Geranium Oil (in the 1800s) and is often blended with the more expensive Rose oils. This oil was and still is used in traditional Indian medicine.

PATCHOULI
Note: Base

Patchouli is effective for combating nervous disorders and helping with dandruff, sores, acne, skin irritations and acne. The specific properties include use as an antidepressant, anti-inflammatory, fungicidal, nerving, stimulating, and tonic agent. The aroma of Patchouli will impart a calming musky sweetness to blends.

Botanical Name: *Pogostemon cablin*
Plant Part: Leaves
Extraction Method: Steam
Origin: Papua New Guinea
Strength of Aroma: Medium

Blends Well with: Sandalwood, Bergamot, Cedarwood, Rose, Orange, Cassia, Myrrh, and Clary Sage

Aromatic Scent: Warm, earthy aroma with fresh fruit-like tones

History: Indian shawls were impregnated with Patchouli, and they them became popular in Europe in the 1900s. In 1960, hippies used it for perfume oil and incense because the strong aroma masks marijuana.

PETITGRAIN
Note: Middle

Petitgrain is known to have uplifting properties and has long been used to calm anger and reduce stress. It has been used in the skin care industry for acne and oily skin; it can also be used as a deodorizing agent.

Botanical Name: *Petitgrain bigarde*
Plant Part: Leaves and twigs
Extraction Method: Steam
Origin: France
Strength of Aroma: Medium

Blends Well with: Bergamot, Cedarwood, Clary Sage, Geranium, Lavender, Lime, Jasmine, Neroli, Orange, Palmarosa, Rosemary, Rosewood, Sandalwood, and Ylang Ylang.

Aromatic Scent: Orange blossoms with a bitter, woody and herbaceous undertone

History: Originally this oil was created from the green unripe oranges when they were still the size of cherries; hence the French term *Petitgrain*, which means "little grain." This proved uneconomical and so the oil began being extracted from the leaves and twigs of the orange tree instead.

PEPPERMINT
Note: Top

Peppermint is an invigorating and cooling oil, which has a warming effect also. It is an ingredient in toothpaste and cosmetics and can be helpful for cough, cold, and digestive problems. It is ideal for use to benefit colds, flu, headaches, and mental fatigue. It helps clear the mind and allows you to focus.

Botanical Name: *Mentha arvensis*
Plant Part: Flowering herb
Extraction Method: Steam
Origin: Nepal
Strength of Aroma: Medium to strong

Blends Well with: Basil, Bergamot, Cedarwood, Eucalyptus, Lemon, Lime, Mandarin, Marjoram, Pine, Rosemary, and Thyme.

Aromatic Scent: Sharp, penetrating mint scent based on its high menthol content. The sweetness of the vapor makes it easy to see why it is such a common flavoring and scenting agent.

History: Peppermint and its name have its roots in Greek mythology. Pluto, god of the dead, fell in love with Minthe, herself a beautiful nymph. Pluto's goddess wife Persephone became jealous and turned Minthe into a plant, but out of respect for her beauty, she ensured that she would have a wonderful and fragrant aroma.

PINE
Note: Top / Middle

A powerful antiseptic, Pine is used as part of detergents and house cleaning products. It will help detoxify the body and is ideal for steam inhalation for respiratory ailments. It is warming and soothing for tired muscles.

Botanical Name: *Pinus sylvestris*
Plant Part: Twigs and needles
Extraction: Steam distillation
Origin: Russia and Austria
Strength of Aroma: Strong

Blends Well with: Lavender, Lemon, Eucalyptus, Frankincense, Juniper, Neroli, Rose, and Ylang Ylang

Aromatic Scent: Sweet, fresh Christmas tree-like aroma

History: Originating in Russia and Austria, Pine spread to different parts of the world.

ROSE
Note: Middle

Rose is one of the most expensive oils but the benefits make it worth having a small bottle around. (It can be bought in 3 percent Jojoba, which is still expensive but unreasonable.) Calming and comforting, Rose helps to dispel tension. It is ideal for sleeplessness, and it improves circulation. It helps ease discomfort associated with pre-menstruation, menstruation, and menopause. Rose is well-loved oil but is expensive because of its extraction method. A blend of Geranium and Palmarosa smells similar to Rose and is not as expensive.

Botanical Name: *Rosa damascene*
Plant Part: Petals
Extraction: Steam distillation
Origin: India, Indonesia
Strength of Aroma: Strong

Blends Well with: Bergamot, Chamomile, Clary Sage, Geranium, Lavender, Jasmine, Neroli, Orange, Patchouli, and Sandalwood

Aromatic Scent: Very rich, sweet-floral, scent

History: No other flower in documented history has been more exalted in literature and mythology and used in sacred purposes as the Rose. In ancient art, the rose blossoms symbolized beauty, love, youth, and immortality. The word *rosa* comes from the Greek word *rodon* (red). It was prized in Babylon, Assyria, China, Rome, and Greece. These cultures were aware of the healing powers found in Rose.

ROSEMARY
Note: Top / Middle

Strengthening invigorating oil useful for low blood pressure, Rosemary helps stimulate weak memory and enhance concentration. It may relieve systems associated with digestive upsets and muscle tension. It can be part of a blend to help with dandruff and promotes mental alertness.

Botanical Name: *Rosmarinus officinalis*
Plant Part: Herb
Extraction Method: Steam
Origin: France
Strength of Aroma: Medium to strong

Blends Well with: Basil, Bergamot, Cedarwood, Frankincense, Ginger, Lavender, Lemon, Orange, and Peppermint

Aromatic Scent: A fresh, strong, woody, Balsamic scent

History: Because Rosemary grows in proximity to the sea, its name means Dew of the Sea. Its leaves were traditionally burned in hospitals to purify the air. Rosemary was used as incense by the ancient Romans. According to legend, Mary sheltered the baby Jesus under a Rosemary bush. Rosemary was used by the ancient Egyptians in their cleansing rituals. Napoleon was more interesting in using it for focusing the mind and was reputed to use large quantities of Rosemary cologne.

Cautions: Not suitable for people with epilepsy or high blood pressure. Avoid in pregnancy. Might antidote homeopathic remedies.

SAGE
Note: Top

The therapeutic properties of Sage Essential Oil are as an anti-inflammatory, antiseptic, astringent, digestive, diuretic, insecticide, laxative and a tonic.

Botanical Name: *Salvia officinalis*
Plant Part: Leaves
Extraction Method: Steam
Origin: Croatia
Strength of Aroma: Strong

Blends Well with: Bergamot, Lavender, Lemon, and Rosemary

Aromatic Scent: Sage has a spicy, sharp, and very herbaceous scent. It is referred to as having a penetrating and powerful aroma.

History: The Chinese believed Sage cured sterility and the Romans believed it cured just about everything. The Latin word *salvare* means "heal" or "save." During the Middle Ages, Sage was a popular ingredient of many nerve tonics and the actual herb was used to clean gums.

SANDALWOOD
Note: Base

Sandalwood oil is usually expensive. Time quality oil is hard to come by because it comes from a 20-50 year old tree, which is why the price varies so much between seasons. Use Sandalwood to combat bronchitis, chapped and dry skin, depression, laryngitis, oily skin, scars sensitive skin, stress, and stretch marks. It also has historical applications as an aid in meditation for religious ceremonies.

Botanical Name: *Santalum spicatum*
Plant Part: Wood
Extraction Method: Steam
Origin: Australia (WA)
Strength of Aroma: Medium

Blends Well with: Most oils: Rose, Clove, Lavender, Geranium, Vetiver, Patchouli, Jasmine, Bergamot, Clary Sage, Coriander, Cypress, Fennel, Frankincense, Myrrh, Palmarosa, Pepper, and Peppermint

Aromatic Scent: Sandalwood East Indian is a rich, balsamic, sweet fragrance with delicate wood notes that add to its reputation as luxurious and exquisite oil. It is a prized ingredient in perfumes and is especially appreciates by men.

History: The documented use of Sandalwood goes back 4000 years to India, Egypt, Greece, and Rome. Many temples and structures were built from Sandalwood and the Egyptians used it in embalming.

TEA TREE
Note: Top / Middle

Tea Tree is best known as a very powerful immune stimulant. It can help to fight off infectious. Used in vapor therapy, it can help with colds, measles, sinusitis, and viral infections. For skin and hair, Tea Tree has been used to combat acne, oily skin, head lice, and dandruff. Tea Tree is "first aid" in a bottle.

Botanical Name: *Melaleuca alternifolia*
Plant Part: Leaves
Extraction Method: Steam
Origin: Australia
Strength of Aroma: Medium to strong

Blends Well with: Cinnamon, Clary Sage, Clove, Geranium, Lavender, Lemon, Myrrh, Nutmeg, Rosewood, Rosemary, and Thyme

Aromatic Scent: A fresh, antiseptic and medicinal scent

History: Tea tree has a long history of use within the field of aromatherapy. In World War II, the producers and the cutters of Tea Tree were exempt from military service until enough Essential Oil had been accumulated.

THYME
Note: Middle

Thyme is used in inhalation to reduce the symptoms of cough and bronchitis. Medicinally, thyme is used for respiratory infections in the form of a tincture, tisane, and salve, or by steam inhalation. It is a powerful healer used for skin infections and dermatitis.

Botanical Name: *Thymus vulgaris*
Plant Part: Herb
Extraction Method: CO_2
Origin: France
Strength of Aroma: Medium

Blends Well with: Cinnamon, Clary Sage, Clove, Geranium, Lavender, Lemon, Myrrh, Nutmeg, Rosewood, Rosemary, and Thyme

Aromatic Scent: Sweet, warm, and herbaceous

History: Before the advent of modern antibiotics, Thyme was used to medicate bandages. It has also been shown to be effective against the fungus that commonly infects toenails.

VETIVER
Note: Base

Vetivert is deeply relaxing and comforting oil with a strong dirt-like aroma. It is used as a base note in perfumery (usually oriental fragrances) and aromatherapy applications. Vetiver is sometime known as the oil of tranquility because of its ability to strengthen the nervous system. With antifungal and antibacterial properties, it may also be used in treatment of acne and minor cuts.

Botanical Name: *Vetiveria zizanoides*
Plant Part: Root
Extraction Method: Steam
Origin: Java
Strength of Aroma: Strong

Blends Well with: Cedarwood, Chamomile, Frankincense, Ginger, Jasmine, Juniper, Lavender, Lemongrass, Patchouli, Rose, Sandalwood, Spikenard, Vanilla, and Ylang Ylang

Aromatic Scent: Vetiver has an earthy, woody scent characteristic of most Essential Oils derived from roots in the earth. It also has a rich, sweetly satisfying note that is both warm and masculine.

History: In Georgian times, it was fashionable to have perfume handkerchief fragranced with Vetiver; it was used in traditional Indian households.

YLANG YLANG
Note: Base

Ylang Ylang is an Essential Oil that helps lift moods and is believed to lessen inhibition. With a very sweet exotic scent, it is a reputed aphrodisiac, a powerful stimulant, and euphoric. It can be used as a sedative and has a regulating effect on the nervous system. A general cleaner for skin and hair, Ylang Ylang helps prevent dandruff. It is been used extensively in perfumes and cosmetic applications.

Botanical Name: *Cananga odorata*
Plant Part: Flower extraction
Method: Steam
Origin: France
Strength of Aroma: Medium

Blends Well with: Bergamot, Grapefruit, Lavender, Neroli, Rosewood, and Sandalwood

Aromatic Scent: Sweet, exotic, floral scent that is one of the most sought after aromas.

History: In Indonesia, Ylang Ylang flower petals are strewn upon the bed of newlywed couples. Ylang Ylang was a popular ingredient of hair preparations in Europe.

Cautions: Can cause sensitivity on some people; excessive use may lead to headaches and nausea

Conclusion

Conclusion

As you can see, the world of Aromatherapy and Essential Oils is amazing and diverse. I love that you can create your own products so simply and that you can adjust them to your individual likes and dislikes.

Using Essential Oil and making natural products for you, your family, and friends are great ways to save money and benefit from the therapeutic properties at the same time.

I hope you have enjoyed learning and making your own natural products. This is only the only the beginning of your enjoyment of using Essential Oils for every day.

The Essential 5: How to Make Natural Products Using 5 Essential Oils or Less. Over 200 Simple and Effective Recipes was created to give you an understanding of aromatherapy, enable you to save money, and make products quickly and simply.

BIOGRAPHY

Tina is business owner, graphic/web designer and author with over 20 years combined knowledge in business, time management, training, and design. Joining this with her understanding and passion for Essential Oils and Aromatherapy, Tina has created for your enjoyment, The Essential 5.

She believes in living life with passion and determination and loves helping people create simple effective solutions to daily life and this is the basis of The Essential 5.

To complement this book Tina is currently writing Maximize your Essential Worth: A Guide to Understanding Your True Value and Creating Success in All Areas of Life.

Tina also designs website for clients and assists them in achieving success in their given fields, she understands that marketing on the internet is so much more that putting up a template base website, instead she strives to create individual plans for each clients needs.

As an energetic and positive author, designer and mum, Tina is a dynamic person, allowing her life experience to shine through while giving practical and simple effective solutions that are fun and inspiring to learn and use.

These days Tina can be found helping people create their own products, create balance in their lives, and find the true Essential Worth.

Tina Fletcher was born in Bargo, New South Wales, but has lived most of her life in Queensland. She has lived in various places, first with her parents and siblings, then by herself moving with work commitments, and later with her husband.

Living in Mackay when her marriage broke down, she stayed for a little while and then decided to move to a smaller country town for the lifestyle she wanted for her children. Tina now lives in Ayr, Queensland, with her five children.

A born entrepreneur, Tina has shown her business drive from a early age where at 17 she ran a chicken takeaway; from there she did three years in the Army. On leaving the military she married and traveled around the world for a couple of years.

Upon returning to Australia, she started her own graphics business which she ran for many years. At this time she found her love of Essential Oils and showing people how to use them and benefit from them.

While looking after her family Tina tried to always maintain her balance in life and has endeavored to show other to do the same.

INDEX

1 Minute Stress Buster, 146
10% Essential Oil Blend, 158
10% Pure Oil Blend, 154
100% Pure Essential Oil Blend, 153, 157
After Sun Gel, 109
Air Conditioners, 69
Air Conditioners Filters, 69
Air Fresher Spray, 57, 67
All Purpose Cleanser, 59, 68
Aloe Gera Gel, 38
Antiseptic Cream, 98, 101
Ants, 69
Apricot Kernel Oil, 35
Aromatherapy, 244
Aromatherapy History, 246
Arthritis, 124
Athlete's Foot, 109
Atomisers, 145
Atomizers, 45
Avocado Oil, 35

Base Cream, 39
Base Note, 30
Base Oil, 39
Base Oil Properties, 35
Base Oils, 34
Base Products, 38
Basil Essential Oil, 250
Bath Bombs, 145, 159, 233
Bath Oil, 146
Bath Oil - Dissolving, 160, 235
Bath Oils, 234
Bath Salts, 145, 155, 161, 236
Bathing, 45, 145
Bathrooms, 70
Bed Time Ritual, 146
Benches, 71
Bergamot Essential Oil, 251
Bicarb, 39
Bicarb Shaker, 58, 70
Black Pepper Essential Oil, 252
Blend, 13, 45
Blisters, 110
Blisters (from Burns), 110
Body Oil, 155, 161, 173, 237
Boiling, 48
Boils, 110
Bottles, 26
Brass, 71
Burn Gel - minor burns, 102
Buying Essential Oils, 26

Candles, 147
Car Sickness, 125
Car Windows, 72
Carpet Stains, 72
Carpets, 72
Cautions, 32
Cedarwood Essential Oil, 253
Chamomile Essential Oil, 18, 254
Chapped Lips, 102
Chicken Pox, 111
Chrome, 73
Cigarette Burns, 111
Cinnamon Essential Oil, 255
Citronella Essential Oil, 256
Clary Sage Essential Oil, 257
Cleanser, Skin, 169, 174
Cleansing Oil, 175
Clove Essential Oil, 258
Cobwebs, 73
Cockroaches, 73
Coffee stains, 74
Cold Sores, 103
Common Ailments, 97
Compress, 46, 147
Conditioner, Eggy, 194
Conditioners, 193
Cooking Smells, 73
Cost Benefits, 21
Craddle Cap, 112
Cupboards, 74
Curtains, 74
Cuts, 113, 126
Cutting Boards, 74
Cypress Essential Oil, 259

Dark Hair Brightener, 195
Deodorant, 221, 224
Dermatitis - Babies, 113
Detergent or Pure Soap, 40
Diffusers, 47, 150
Direct application, 46, 147
Dishwashing Liquid, 61, 76
Disinfectant, 60, 75
Drains, 77
Drawers, 77
Drinking Glasses, 80
Dryer, 77

Ea de Toilette, 226
Eau de Cologne, 220, 225
Eczema, 114
Eczema - Babies, 113
Eczema Gel, 103

Effective Applications, 45
Eggs, 40
Epson Salt, 40
Essential Oil Properties, 249
Essential Oils, 248
Eucalyptus Essential Oil, 260
Evening Primrose, 35
Exercise, 148
Eye Glasses, 78

Face Mask, 172, 176
Face Spray, 156, 162, 177, 238
Fair Hair Brightener, 195
First Aid, 97
Floor Cleaner, 62, 78
Fly Screens, 79
Foot Odor, 127
Footbath, 46, 148
Fragrant Oils, 27
Frankincense Essential Oil, 261
Fridges, 79
Frizz Away Treatment, 196

Geranium Essential Oil, 17, 262
Gift Ideas, 231
Ginger Essential Oil, 263
Glass, 80
Grapefruit Essential Oil, 264
Grapeseed Oil, 35
Grazes, 115
Grime Cleaner, 70
Grout, 80

Hair Care, 187, 192
Hair Gel, 196
Hair Mousse, 202
Hair Spray, 197
Hangover, 127
Hay fever, 128
Hayfever, 115
Head Lice, 116
Head Lice Daily Spray, 118, 200
Head Lice Hair Treatment, 105, 199
Head Lice Shampoo, 116, 198
Head Lice Treatment, 117
Headaches, 106, 128
Hiccups, 114
Hives, 118
Hot Oil Treatment, 190, 201
House Cleaning, 51
Humidifiers, 46, 148

Influenza, 129
Inhalation, 47, 149
Insect Bites, 104, 119
Insect Repellent, 63, 81, 130

Ironing Spray, 82
Itching, 131

Jasmine Essential Oil, 19, 265
Jojoba Oil, 36
Journal or Diary, 149
Juniper Berry Essential Oil, 266
Juniper Essential Oil, 266

Labels, 49, 82
Laundry, 82
Lavender Essential Oil, 17, 267
Lavender Sachets, 238
Leave in Conditioner, 191, 202
Lemon Essential Oil, 17, 268
Light Bulbs, 83
Lime Essential Oil, 269
Liquid Soap Mix, 41

Making Your Own, 43
Marjoram Essential Oil, 270
Massage, 47, 149
Mediation, 151
Microwaves, 83
Middle Note, 29, 30
Mildew, 84
Mirrors, 64, 84
Morning Sickness, 131
Mosquitoes, 85
Moths, 85
Mould, 86
Music, 151
Myrrh Essential Oil, 271

Nappy Rash, 120
Natural, 25
Natural Conditioner, 189, 193
Natural Shampoo, 188, 204
Nausea, 132
Night Cream, 172, 179
No chemicals, 24
Notes, 13

Oil burners, 150
Oils burners, 47
Olive Oil, 36
Orange Essential Oil, 272
Osteoarthritis, 124
Oven Cleaner, 86

Palmarosa Essential Oil, 273
Paper Mache Gifts, 239
Patchouli Essential Oil, 274
Peppermint Essential Oil, 276
Perfume, 222, 228
Perfumed Body Oil, 219, 224

– Index –

Perfumed Soap, 218, 229
Perfumed Talc, 219, 230
Perfumes Liquid Soap, 227
Petitgrain Essential Oil, 275
Pine Essential Oil, 277
Play Dough, 242
Polishing, 87
Pots and Pans, 87
Properties, 13
Psoriasis Hair Treatment, 203
Pure Essential Oil Blend, 153
Pure Essential Oils, 27
Pure Soap (Liquid Soap Mix), 40

Quick Relief, 150

Rashes, 120, 133
Recipe, 13
Refreshing & Uplifting Blend, 144, 153
Refrigerators, 79
Relaxation Release Blend, 144, 153
Rheumatoid Arthritis, 124
Room Deodorizer, 87
Room Spray, 150
Rose Essential Oil, 278
Rosemary Essential Oil, 279
Rust, 88

Safflower Oil, 36
Sage Essential Oil, 280
Salt, 41
Sand Flies, 121
Sandalwood Essential Oil, 281
Scented Beads, 239
Scented Drink Coaster, 241
Scented Mobiles, 240
Scented Pendants, 240
Shampoos, 204
Shaving Rash, 121
Shine Rinse, 191, 206
Shoes, 88
Shower, 47, 88, 150
Shower Head, 89

Sinus Blend, 106, 112
Sinusitis, 134
Skin care Moisturizer, 171, 178
Skin Toner, 170, 179
Soap, 89
Spiders, 89
Stainless Steel Cleaner, 90
Steaming, 48
Sterilizers, 48
Stickers, 90
Straightening Hair Spray, 206
Stress Buster Blend, 144, 153
Sunburn, 107, 121
Sunflower Oil, 36
Surface Spray, 65, 91
Sweet Almond Oil, 37

Talc, 219, 230
Taps, 92
Tea stain cups, 74
Tea Tree Essential Oil, 18, 282
Thyme Essential Oil, 283
Tile Grout, 92
Tiles, 92
Toilet, 93
Toilet Deodorizer, 93
Top Note, 29, 30
Travel Sickness, 134

Vetiver Essential Oil, 284
Vinegar, 41
Vinegar Spray, 66, 93

Warts, 135
Washing Up Liquid, 94
Wheatgerm Oil, 37
Window Sills, 95
Windows, 64, 95
Windows - Frost Free, 95
Wounds, 122

Ylang Ylang Essential Oil, 19, 285

Contact Information

Email Tina at: tina@tinafletcherdesigns.com

Mail to Tina at: P.O. Box 478, Ayr Qld 4807

For General Inquires or to

Book Tina to speak at your event:

www.TinaFletcher.com.au

Tina's Website links

Tina Fletcher Designs: For all your Designs Service in One Place –

www.TinaFletcherDesigns.com

The Essential 5 – *www.TheEssential5.com*

Maximizing your Essential Worth – *www.EssentialWorth.com*

www.ingramcontent.com/pod-product-compliance
Lightning Source LLC
Chambersburg PA
CBHW071658160426
43195CB00012B/1511